Transforming Healthcare Education

Teaching Ethics
Across the American Educational Experience

Dominic P. Scibilia, Editor

Transforming Healthcare Education

Applied Lessons Leading to Deeper Moral Reflection

Edited by Philip C. Scibilia and
Dominic P. Scibilia

Series edited by Dominic P. Scibilia

ROWMAN & LITTLEFIELD
Lanham • Boulder • New York • London

Published by Rowman & Littlefield
An imprint of The Rowman & Littlefield Publishing Group, Inc.
4501 Forbes Boulevard, Suite 200, Lanham, Maryland 20706
www.rowman.com

6 Tinworth Street, London SE11 5AL, United Kingdom

Copyright © 2020 by Philip C. Scibilia

All rights reserved. No part of this book may be reproduced in any form or by any electronic or mechanical means, including information storage and retrieval systems, without written permission from the publisher, except by a reviewer who may quote passages in a review.

British Library Cataloguing in Publication Information Available

Library of Congress Cataloging-in-Publication Data Available

Library of Congress Control Number: 2020930426

ISBN: 978-1-4758-4592-1 (cloth)
ISBN: 978-1-4758-4593-8 (pbk.)
ISBN: 978-1-4758-4594-5 (electronic)

Contents

Series Preface — vii
Dominic P. Scibilia

Foreword — xi
Thomas F. Zimmerman

Introduction — xiii
Philip C. Scibilia

1 Bioethics Matters: Clinical Ethics at the Bedside — 1
  Jeanne Kerwin

2 A Model for Training Bioethics Consultants (for the In-House Seminar or Regional Workshop) — 15
  Jeanne Kerwin

3 Drinking Stories: A Narrative Approach to Teaching the Neuroethics of Addiction — 29
  Katie Grogan

4 Calling for Racial Equity Training in Medical School Curriculum — 43
  Kirk Johnson

5 Racial Equity: A Pedagogical Model — 53
  Kirk Johnson

6 Hearing the Voice of the Sufferer: The Moral Compass of the Healthcare Professional — 63
  Gaetana Kopchinsky

7	Epigogy: The Education of Humanity: The Psychology of Pain as It Affects the Human Condition *Gaetana Kopchinsky*	73
8	Epilogue *Philip C. Scibilia*	93

About the Authors   95

Series Preface
Dominic P. Scibilia, PhD

What is the American social compact on education? From Jefferson's vision of a public education that forms and informs a democratic citizenry to current education secretary in the Trump administration Betsy DeVos's call to ease church-state regulations regarding education, proposing $5 billion of public money to fund private and religious education (as a means of providing fair access to better schools than implied substandard public schools), the current state of our national educational narrative is often framed by claims in conflict or claims that public education is deficient.

A great deal of the debate regarding the American educational experience since 1987 has focused on deficiencies—what students cannot do. Many works by commentators like Rudolf Flesch (1986), Allan Bloom (1987), and Erika Christakis (*The Atlantic* 2017) have critically observed that students cannot read or write, or are unable to distinguish right from wrong, or that the trends in national public educational policy encourage a dystopian view of public schools.

In response to the conflicting claims about education in America, pedagogues propose whole curricula, design lessons, and implement assessments framed with SMART goals, backward curriculum design, summative or formative measurements of learning, and professional learning communities as antidotes for what ails schools from kindergarten through graduate schools.

The past thirty years in American education feel like an extended autumn. The debaters and conversation partners look too often like people witnessing the browning of the American public educational experience—as if it has been dying. Caught in the melancholy that sometimes accompanies autumn, catching us up in a deep appreciation for the beauty of the season and the advent of death, we miss the seeding that is occurring. Our children in public schools as much as in independent or religious schools are indeed learning to read, write, reason critically, create, and know right from wrong—imagine morally.

Insight into the state of our national educational narrative, the social compact we have with our children regarding their education and with each other regarding the forming and informing of democratic citizens, rises from the witness of the patriots who teach especially ethics.

The series *Teaching Ethics across the American Educational Experience* gives us pause to consider the moral seeding underway throughout American schools. Indeed, students are learning how to distinguish right from wrong, to engage reason, emotion and imagination when acting as moral agents. During the spring of 2018, Tom Koerner, vice president for Rowman & Littlefield, encouraged me to raise the witnesses whose words and works provide evidence of effective learning, of the seeding of the moral imagination for future citizens.

MARCH 14, 2018

It has been a month since the shootings and killing of seventeen adults and students at Marjory Stoneman Douglas High School in Parkland, Florida. The front page of *The New York Times* frames the infancy narrative of the student social movement #NeverAgain. Like many student movements from around the world (from Colombia, Mexico City, and Taiwan to the call for public education in Valparaiso, Chile), Parkland High School students call for social change.

Broadcast news services witness the national growth of #NeverAgain as the Parkland students call for a national walkout from school at 10 a.m. today for a seventeen-minute memorial to those who died on February 14. Online and television cameras broadcast pictures of students and adults from Parkland, Atlanta, Decatur, Washington D.C., New York City and as the Central and Mountain time zones reach 10 a.m. from Chicago, Littleton in Colorado, and schools in Idaho. They walk out from classes with and without administrative permission.

Adolescents soon to break in on adulthood express ideas like civic responsibility, social reform, political will, civil disobedience, constitutional rights in conflict, and legislative change. They announce their advent as voters. How did those young citizens arrive at moments of political engagement? What stirred their social and moral imaginations—seeing visions of a good society in contrast to their experiences of a flawed society? How did they cultivate abilities to assess critically the functions and dysfunctions within our American political systems?

Someone designed and implemented educational experiences that proved to be effective learning moments in social ethics. The evidence for effective learning in that student movement is not measured by a test score; rather, the evidence comes in the students' applications of their moral imaginations to social questions. Look at how they act, at what they do. As their moral imaginations provoke civic engagement, students become the sort of citizens that advocates for public education, from Jefferson to Dewey to Weingarten, hope would graduate from American schools.

MARCH 14, 2019

There are teachers from kindergarten through senior year of high school, from undergraduate classrooms to postgraduate professional seminars and corporate committees who design and implement ethics instruction and assess the effectiveness of learning ethics. Those teachers have been responding consistently since the late 1980s to the caustic criticism that a moral vacuum exists in American schools: that Johnny and Jane cannot tell right from wrong as well as read.

Teaching Ethics across the American Educational Experience celebrates the commitment of educators who teach ethics. The contributors in each of the five books in this series take time to write about how students are learning ethics—how instructors teach ethics. It is an unusual writing for teachers. Few preschool and K–12 teachers receive the time to reflect critically on and write about instruction, especially teaching ethics. The demand for scholarship in higher learning rarely considers works seated in a critical reflection on instructional design and implementation—practical works rather than the intellectual kind.

In *Teaching Ethics across the American Educational Experience*, teachers take the time to consider ethical instruction and its effectiveness. They present models for ethics instruction and learning from kindergarten through professional life. Lesson plans, integrative plans across a school's curriculum, templates for implementation, and means of learning assessment populate five teacher-friendly, student-centered, practical monographs. The series' goals encourage teachers to pause and in that critical contemplative space consider integrating ethics into their American students' educational experiences.

These five texts call readers to respond to our witness—the instructional experiences that invite students to be citizens carrying out the American experiment. *Teaching Ethics across the American Educational Experience* offers the witness of administrators, teachers, parents, the teachers of teachers, and students who will stir moral imaginations to design and implement learning ethics, to open effectively American hearts, souls, and minds. We raise a witness to the current state of our national educational social compact.

Brian Gatens, superintendent of the Emerson Public Schools District in New Jersey (Emerson, New Jersey), opens a literary space wherein administrators and teachers model integrating ethics instruction within a social-emotional learning framework—education attending to the whole child.

Kristen Hawley Turner (Drew University) convenes a community of educators from elementary school through graduate educational studies for dynamic conversations on the ethical dimensions of teaching digital literacy.

Jane Bleasdale and Julie Sullivan's (University of San Francisco) volume invites middle and high school teachers to offer models of teaching ethics (stirring self and social awareness that leads to civic agency) in public and independent high schools.

Daniel Wueste (Clemson University) gathers a symposium of university faculty (many of whom are members of the Society for Ethics across the Curriculum) proposing models for teaching ethics across undergraduate studies.

Philip Scibilia (medical humanist) calls together graduate school professionals who offer prescient instructional models for teaching narrative ethics within a medical humanist praxis across healthcare curricula.

Foreword

Healthcare has been and remains caught in a major paradigm shift. A paraphrase of a quote often ascribed to Mahatma Gandhi, *There go my followers. I am their leader. I had better hurry*, describes the medical humanities relative to these changes. Disruptive technologies, from imaging diagnostics and biotherapeutics to mobility apps, and emerging new players such as Amazon and Microsoft move forward, far outpacing attention to the human dimensions of care.

While healthcare changes spin ever faster, the polar moral axis remains a constant. The *north pole* is the duty of beneficence, the *south pole* nonmaleficence. The professional human duty is to provide beneficial care balanced with the duty to do no harm. That duty calls healthcare providers to carefully and respectfully balance the scales of benefit and risk. Virtue ethics principles such as beneficence and nonmaleficence, in addition to justice and respect for persons, should balance the values of scientific and technological advances in healthcare.

Dating back to the 1980s, a number of initiatives have been attempted to operationalize the human dimensions of healthcare. Advanced directives express who should act as a surrogate decision-maker and what interventions are accepted. Respect for autonomy and self-determination in clinical decision-making undergird medical practice. Confidentiality of personal health information and informed consent, an extension of the principle of autonomy, affirm the dignity and rights of the patient as person. The Institutional Review Board provides insight into the expanded role of ethics in research, publication, and continuing professional education.

Over a four-decade career journey, I have been privileged to observe and participate in the U.S. healthcare enterprise in a variety of roles and from a diversity of perspectives: academia, healthcare professional associations, healthcare professional education, research, and healthcare policy. I witnessed the transition from not-for-profit hospitals to the dominance of for-profit medical centers and systems. As a student of the impact of technologies on healthcare practice, I experienced the effects of commercial interest on policy, education, and clinical practice.

During my career journey, I have had the privilege of working on a variety of projects with Dr. Philip C. Scibilia, the editor for this work. The chapters that follow bring attention and provide needed resources for the continued development of the interdisciplinary medical humanities field of study and practice. The guiding spirit for this book (and one for the series of which the book is a part) is the seminal bioethicist Edmund Daniel Pellegrino. Dr. Pellegrino, like his peers Paul Ramsey and Allen Verhey, admonished healthcare as a moral enterprise.

The contributors to this work encourage healthcare professionals to engage in intellectual and moral virtue and provide care in a humanitarian way. The patient as a human being is the focus of care. The authors assembled for this important publication teach within education and healthcare with widely recognized medical humanities programs. They serve in the company of leaders in this expanding academic discipline, in clinical care and in research. The chapters included in this volume focus much-needed attention on, advance ideas for, and—most important—advance actions toward a twenty-first-century expression of ethical healthcare.

Thomas F. Zimmerman

Distinguished Senior Fellow, Shar School of Policy and Government

George Mason University

Introduction
Philip C. Scibilia, DMH

This book clarifies current deliberations on ethics and its application to healthcare in the twenty-first century. The contributors give particular attention to race, equity, the patient as a person, especially the voice of the pain sufferer, and addiction treatment.

The word "ethics," in classical Greek, means *the beliefs of the people*, their study of what is right and good in human conduct and the justification of such claims. Without a doubt, this task is not simply about setting up a list of rights and wrongs. Rather, it is a discussion, a process that helps tease out the real issues and find and teach ethical solutions to complex practical problems. The centrality of the patient is of prime consideration in this book, and the health of the individual patient is the first consideration in the teaching considerations discussed.

Applied ethics in healthcare may have lost sight of what traditional ethics was trying to accomplish: a good life for good people over a lifetime in society with others. The conversation partners in this volume put biomedical ethics into that perspective and contribute to the development of a truly comprehensive approach to healthcare ethics. On the practical level, we provide structures that integrate the givers' ethical perspectives.

But there persists a gap and significant perception differences among healthcare providers' learning environments and actual professional situations. Teaching ethics over the last sixty years, healthcare professionals have struggled with dehumanizing tendencies created by the unprecedented success of modern medicine. Therefore, teaching ethics and healthcare provider's values is important to bridging this gap. In *Transforming Healtcare Education*, we offer pedagogical models that connect a good life for people in a practice of healthcare advancing without sufficient time for critical moral reflection.

Healthcare practice and healthcare education today are the victims of their own success. The science and technology that have brought enormous advances in curing disease, relieving suffering, and extending longevity have also outstripped medicine's moral bearing and overwhelmed the human dimensions of caring, learning, and ethics

Medical technology has shifted attention to machines rather than patients: growing incentives to put profits above patients, a biomedical reductionism that attends to pain but not suffering. Doctors become disease detectives and patients become repositories of disease. Progress in biomedicine has also generated a great deal of moral uncertainty and ethical conflict. Problematic issues arise, such as the protection of research subjects, the goals of healthcare, the definition of death, the rights of patients, the cessation of treatment, the meaning of illness, and the distribution of healthcare resources. Technological trends broaden the portfolio of ethical concerns well beyond the traditional confines of the physician-patient relationship.

The chapters that follow present the framework for ordering and analyzing contemporary health issues. They discuss dedicated, interactive competency-based teaching suggestions vital to support learning on how to integrate ethical thinking with competencies in patient care.

In the first two chapters, Jeanne Kerwin calls for the training of bioethics consultants who offer patients, their families, and medical staff the highest quality of bioethical analysis and conflict resolution. The second chapter breaks open an instructional model (an in-house seminar or regional workshop) of the needed training in bioethical analysis and conflict resolution.

In "Drinking Stories: A Narrative Approach to Teaching the Neuroethics of Addiction," Katie Grogan invites readers to a one-hour workshop in which the internal medicine residents at one academic medical institution examine the neuroethics of addiction through a narrative lens reading of "Big Blonde," a 1929 short story by Dorothy Parker.

Kirk Johnson, in chapter 4, gives pedagogical witness that testifies to the need for race equity training in the medical school curriculum. He follows that witness with an instructional model that defuses tension between doctors discussing race and privilege and works to bridge the gap between the quality of healthcare offered to black and white people.

In the last two chapters, Gaetana Kopchinsky presses the teachers of healthcare professionals to design and offer courses that address the management and semantics of pain as told by people in pain. She, then, offers a medical humanities seminar in which healthcare professionals consider what the voices of the vulnerable tell about the impact of pain on the human condition.

Chapter 1

Bioethics Matters: Clinical Ethics at the Bedside

Jeanne Kerwin

The chapter raises a call for providing to patients, families, and healthcare staff the highest quality of bioethical analysis and conflict resolution. We cannot expect anything less than to assure that our patients, their families, and our medical staff have access to a bioethics consultation service that provides educated and trained consultants with expertise and experience in this incredibly important role within all healthcare facilities.

THE CALL FOR TRAINED BIOETHICS CONSULTANTS

Our society, through its governing laws and norms, is organized around our collective ethical perceptions of right and wrong. Our laws protect us from perceived *wrongs* and we learn at an early age from our parents, teachers, religious leaders, and other authority figures what behavior is acceptable and what is not, and what behaviors are punishable within our family structure and within the law. Within our society, most professions operate according to a *code of ethics*, either inherent in its procedures and protocols or written in declarations.

Some professions are regulated by outside authorities; for example, the food and drug industry is regulated by a federal agency to guard the safety of the public. The profession of medicine is basically regulated through professional codes, licensing requirements, and oversight by medical societies and medical boards, as well as State Departments of Health. Constitutional and common law definitions of patients' rights, including the doctrine of informed consent, rights to privacy, rights to autonomous self-determination, rights to protection within research protocols, and specially designed protections for vulnerable populations, drive patient protections.

The vulnerability of patients, the imbalance of power and knowledge between patients and doctors, analysis of harms versus benefits, issues of futility, access to needed treatments, and conflicts among patients, surrogates, and providers about the ethics of a specific intervention or issue give rise to medical ethics dilemmas. Ethical issues involve safeguarding the integrity of the medical profession while equally safeguarding the well-being and autonomy of patients. In the United States, we have developed and evolved a special study of the ethical issues and dilemmas found in the practice of medicine, called *bioethics*.

The use of *bioethics* in the practical world of medicine and hospitalized patients did not emerge until the 1960s and 1970s, when medical knowledge and new technologies drove the quest to extend and prolong life artificially with dialysis machines, mechanical ventilators, artificial feeding tubes, and other interventions applied to save the lives of those who could not support life with their own bodily function. Bioethics developed as a means to apply moral thinking to the practical aspects and decisions involved in clinical encounters with patients and their families.

The landmark case of Karen Ann Quinlan in New Jersey in 1976 illuminated *a right to die* action in the courts (*In re Quinlan* 1976). Karen Ann was a young woman who was diagnosed to be in a state of permanent unconsciousness from a drug overdose, and her life was maintained in the hospital on a mechanical ventilator. *Permanent vegetative state* became a newly coined clinical description for such a state, and few understood the ramifications of modern medicine's ability to create the prolongation of life through artificial means until this case.

The Quinlan case was widely reported in the media across the United States and around the world. Her parents wanted to provide her with a natural death by removing the ventilator in accord with what they believed would be her wishes, but the medical providers refused to withdraw the machine as they believed it would be tantamount to killing her. The New Jersey Supreme Court decision was a call to acknowledge a patient's *right to die* without the constraints of technologies that prolonged life in a nonsapient state.

This concept and the flow of rights that followed from it in other similar cases over the next two decades supported the core principle of respect for the autonomy of patients and their rights to make decisions about medical treatments, even those treatments that were deemed *life-sustaining*. It was the Quinlan judgment that also recommended that hospitals create *ethics committees* for the purpose of resolving such disputes without the need to go through the courts. They opined that these decisions rightfully belong among the patient, family, and physician.

A plethora of cases followed from the Quinlan case, elucidating those rights: rights to refuse artificial feeding; rights of family members and surrogates to use substituted judgment in making decisions for loved ones who no longer had capacity; and the right to refuse medical intervention even for those with nonterminal conditions. These cases make up the body of legal support for the practice and principles of *bioethics* in today's medical environment. New cases and the exploration of contentious issues driven by new technologies and treatments contribute to the clinical dilemmas encountered in bioethics practice and how society gauges right and wrong in medicine.

Bioethics is a dynamic field, changing constantly, as we moved from a paternalistic model of medicine to a patient-centered and autonomy-driven model and continue to add new medical technologies that pose new questions about the limits of medicine as well as new voices that speak out to illuminate injustices and areas of conflicting values.

The study of bioethics involves an in-depth examination of the extensive literature and history describing the beginnings of ethical theories developed from the roots of philosophy and theology and the derivative principles developed from those theories. In the language of bioethics scholars, we refer to these principles, defined by Beauchamp and Childress (1989) in their publication of *Principles of Biomedical Ethics*, as the *cornerstone principles of medical ethics*.

Those well-known principles describe our duty to practice medicine according to the principles of respect for patient autonomy, beneficence, nonmaleficence, and justice. The practice of balancing these principles to assist in deliberations about the decisions made by patients, surrogates, and their medical teams remains a central part of bioethical discussions in the retrospective review of cases, as well as prospective analysis of cases needing resolution.

Bioethics scholars also engage in discussions that involve the macro ethical dilemmas created within the medical care system. Macro issues include such topics as abortion rights, genetic engineering, reproductive technologies, cloning techniques, DNA exploration through the public domain, organ procurement, universal access to medical care, and many other issues that affect our societal views on medicine and patient rights.

Much has been written about this evolution of bioethics and how it has been integrated into the fabric of medicine. *The Birth of Bioethics* by Jonsen (1998) is one such text that illuminates the history and development of bioethics practice as we know it today.

Modern bioethical practice has embraced a movement away from strict principlism as described using the four cornerstones principles toward a more humanitarian approach to the ethical dilemmas. Varying models of ethical analysis described in contemporary literature include the use of virtue ethics, feminist ethics, relational ethics, casuistry, and narrative ethics. The expansion of medical humanities and narrative medicine within the structure of medical education contribute to the use of narrative ethics in many medical facilities where the stories of patients and their providers play an important role in the resolution of conflicts and uncertainty.

With that brief background, this chapter focuses on the application of bioethical analysis and principles in the practice of bioethics in hospitals and other healthcare facilities. A bioethics practice in a hospital or healthcare setting is responsible for responding to the unique clinical situations and disputes that arise in contemporary medical practice. We will examine the critical underpinnings of bioethics education, committee structure and function, and the training and application of consultation services that play a significant role in the success or failure of the practice of bioethics in hospitals and other healthcare facilities.

Although few hospitals, if any, had *bioethics committees* and services at the time of the Karen Ann Quinlan case in 1976, today all hospitals and nursing homes that receive Medicare/Medicaid funding are required by federal regulations to have an interdisciplinary body that provides this service of dispute resolution and most are chartered as *bioethics committees*. In addition, accreditation agencies such as The Joint Commission require hospitals and other healthcare facilities to have a standing mechanism for dispute resolution and ethical practice oversight.

Special recognition programs like the Magnate status for nursing in hospitals focus on nurse participation in bioethics. How hospitals and other facilities comply with these mandates is a much broader challenge that demands closer examination. Bioethics committees and their role and function within a healthcare facility vary greatly in terms of structure, training, responsibilities, and practice.

Bioethics expertise is often not recognized for its positive impact on patients, families, and healthcare professionals as they face the difficult dilemmas created by the complexity of medical treatment decisions. Many bioethics committees exist in hospitals and facilities because of the regulatory mandate but lack recognition as a valued resource for providers and patients within the institution. The structure and makeup of such committees range from committees that have a complete absence of any member with formal academic background and expertise in bioethics to committees run by a full-time salaried bioethicist.

Members of such committees tend to be staff volunteers who have a passion for the subject of bioethics and would be willing participants in further education and training. The structuring of and assigning members to this committee is key to the diversity needed and the willingness and ability of members to engage in ethical deliberation. A committee of diverse healthcare professionals and some assigned community members who are willing to further their education and training have the potential to become a valuable resource to staff and patients in the hospital.

One of the functions of a hospital or healthcare facility's *bioethics committee* is the critical function of providing bioethics consultations for patients, families, and staff to mediate conflicts, and support ethical decision-making and encourage consensus building among the patient, family, and medical professionals. This important role of bioethics is often relegated to those with little or no academic training in bioethics or dispute mediation. The following are some cases where decision-making by a bioethics committee is required:

1. When a decision is made to discharge an end-stage dementia patient to a subacute rehabilitation facility because Medicare will pay for twenty-one days of care, that is clearly the wrong care plan for that patient. Who should address that issue? Does the pressure to get the patient discharged win out over doing the right thing for the patient? Is the length of stay a more important metric than getting the patient into hospice comfort care at the end of life? Is the family requesting rehab for financial reasons? What incentives drive decisions? Who will intervene to raise the issue of advocacy for the patient?
2. When an elderly patient with many chronic disabilities attempts to end her life with an overdose of pain medications, who decides if it is right to honor her choice to refuse life-sustaining treatment?
3. When a chronic dialysis patient refuses to continue with dialysis because his quality of life is unacceptable to him, do we allow him to die? These are common examples of ethical issues that would benefit from a bioethics consultation by those with education and training in bioethics and expertise in navigating the differing opinions and supporting a resolution.

Fortunately, an emerging body of literature has provided guidance for members of bioethics committees about resolving difficult conflicts that arise in medical practice with most of the focus surrounding end-of-life issues. Many books have been written and academic centers offer certificate programs in bioethics for those who wish to pursue further education. Early practitioners who became involved in bioethics in the 1980s and 1990s sometimes chose to pursue academic degrees in bioethics and medical humanities, driven by a thirst for more knowledge and understanding from those who were the leaders and founders of the emerging field.

The history, principles, and models of ethical analysis and dispute resolution gave structure to a new field through academic learning. From the 1980s and 1990s, and continuing today, we have seen a plethora of rich landmark court cases that attracted media attention and court decisions that ignited public passion about the subjects. *End-of-life* choices were challenged, withdrawing artificial life supports was condemned by some, and patients' rights to refuse treatment were catapulted into the public arena.

Religious, political, and academic scholars all weighed in with opinions while medical technological advances continued moving forward at a rapid pace without addressing when such technologies might be ethically challenged. Through discussions and debates about these landmark cases, early bioethics committee members learned about ethical analysis, weighing and balancing principles and examining individual cases and the burdens and benefits of opposing treatment options.

Bioethics scholars from around the country shared experiences and case discussions. In these early bioethics committees, there were ongoing and dynamic educational endeavors to stay current with the changing landscape of medicine and the current ethical issues as they evolved. Committee members learned from each other and the bioethics literature included new and expanded methods of discourse from principle-driven analysis to narrative ethics, casuistry ethics, feminine ethics, and other models that were integrated into the foundational principles of medical ethics.

From the early 1980s when bioethics was a new and challenging field of expertise in healthcare settings to the present mandate for bioethics committees, these committees have been created and are now commonplace in most hospitals. However, the expertise and training of those who sit as members of these committees and perform bioethics consultations remains largely dependent on the individual hospital or facility. Historically there has been no mandate for who should sit on such committees, what their educational background in bioethics should be, and what evaluations and oversight should measure their performance as a bioethics resource.

In 2011, the American Society for Bioethics and Humanities (ASBH) published its report on Core Competencies for Healthcare Ethics Consultation and a companion publication in 2015, *Improving Competencies in Clinical Ethics Consultation: An Education Guide*. Still, there is no mandate to follow, or even to utilize, the Core Competency recommendations as educational information for bioethics committee members and, more importantly, for those performing bioethics consultations.

Because contemporary membership on bioethics committees is determined by each institution according to their unique needs and the priority given to this by their senior leaders, and because there has been no mandate for healthcare facilities to abide by the recommendations and guidance provided in the literature, these committees run the full range of structure and function. Committee membership can be loosely defined and have randomly assigned members who have no background in bioethics and receive no training. Yet other bioethics committees are highly organized and have members who are educated and led by one or two individuals who have academic training and expertise in bioethics.

Based upon in-depth and direct involvement in complex ethical decision-making over the past three decades, it is abundantly clear that *bioethics* matters. Cases that could destroy the integrity of a family, override a patient's clear wishes, manipulate a physician to provide nonbeneficial treatment, or disregard the autonomy of a patient with mental illness all cry out for ethical deliberation, compassionate mediation, and satisfactory resolution.

How, then, do we assure that high-quality bioethics consultation services will be provided to all these vulnerable, distraught patients, the anxious and fearful families, and the physicians who want to act in their best interests? Having a well-trained, experienced, and educated bioethics team is central to a healthcare institution's ability to provide high-quality, compassionate, and humane care to all patients and their families, while preserving the integrity of the medical profession.

Visits to a wide variety of healthcare facilities and teaching bioethics to those who seek or maintain membership on bioethics committees have provided this author with the opportunity to listen to providers describe the makeup of their facility's bioethics committee. Some have all physician department chairs, some rotate members each month to avoid overcommitment on busy staff members, some are limited to administrators and risk management or legal staff, some have open staffing for those who have interest in bioethics, and some have the ideal multidisciplinary membership with a few community members.

Very few have dedicated leadership with academic training and expertise in the practice of bioethics consultation. It is the larger academic medical centers that tend to hire a full-time leader for bioethics with academic training and expertise to direct the bioethics committee and function. Most smaller community hospitals have no academically credentialed leadership for bioethics.

Often bioethics is a low priority for hospital administration and structured only to meet minimum requirements of the Joint Commission and state and federal regulations. Membership is generally volunteered among staff who hold interest in the ethical aspects of medical care. This lends itself to a very wide range of expertise and value for such committees.

The three major recommended functions of a *bioethics committee* by ASBH are (1) policy review and development; (2) education for committee members and facility staff; and (3) bioethics (clinical) consultation services. Some committees function in all three areas, some review cases and the literature, some provide committee education, but many are lacking in the provision of bedside consultation services.

For those that do become involved in consultations, the consultants may lack academic or in-house training on the provision of ethics consultation. As stated in the ASBH Core Competencies, "*It is the clinical subspecialty where unqualified health care ethics consultants (HCEC) have the highest potential to directly harm patients and families as well as others involved in* a consultation . . . the Task Force considers clinical ethics case consultation in which the health care ethics consultant interacts with a patient/family and documents the HCEC activities in the patient's medical record to be where the stakes are often highest"* (ASBH 2011).

Contrary to the recommendations of ASBH to have members of bioethics committees meet certain competencies, and to have at least one member of the consultation service have advanced competencies and training in ethical consultation, a large number of bioethics committees fall far short of these recommendations.

There are three basic models for prospective consultation services: (a) review and opinion by full committee; (b) review and opinion by selected team of two to three members; and (c) one bioethics consultant to review and render opinion. Committees within the healthcare field may have any one of these models or no prospective consultation service. Those who have a consultation service are more at risk when the consultants lack formal training, expertise, and specific credentialing to perform these complex consults where the stakes are high.

When patients, families, and medical providers are faced with moral dilemmas that often involve the life or death of a patient, we should ask why most do not receive high-quality, well-educated, and trained bioethics consultants to assist them in making the most difficult decisions of their lives.

Only starting in 2018 has there been an attempt to *certify* bioethics consultants nationwide (ASBH) through a one-time written exam. The certification process is certainly a move in the right direction but is designed for those with extensive experience in providing ethics consultations (*at least 400 hours of demonstrated clinical ethics experience related to the major domain areas of the HEC-C program content outline within the previous four years*) and is a voluntary process with significant cost.

It begs the question: Will hospitals that put few resources into their bioethics committees create a process to assure their consultants are trained to the level of competency recommended by ASBH and further promote and require certification? The answer is currently unknown. And what do hospitals and other healthcare facilities do to begin a consultation service with untrained staff? How do clinical ethics consultants acquire 400 hours of demonstrated experience without training?

Much more can be said about the current level of competency and administrative support in hospitals and healthcare facilities for their bioethics committees, but suffice is to say that the patients and families who rely on trained, competent, and certified physicians, nurses, and other healthcare practitioners to deliver the best medical care possible should also be assured that those who assist them in the extraordinarily difficult decisions involved in complex medical decisions during serious illness are equally trained, competent, and designated/certified/appointed to do so by the institution in which they practice.

The current autonomy-driven model of medical decision-making is in stark contrast to the paternalistic model of medicine we knew in the 1950s, making difficult decisions about treatment options fall on the plates of patients and their families or surrogates regardless of their abilities to emotionally and intellectually manage the information and choices. The burden and the impact on those who have to make these decisions are significant and often wreak long-term damage to individuals and families (Kerwin 2007, doctoral dissertation). This alone makes the role of bioethics consultation an important and integral part of good medical care.

After almost forty years of growth, development, and recognition of the importance of bioethics in medicine, it has never been more critical to integrate bioethics expertise into best practice standards in the current medical landscape. Bioethical issues continue to include conflicts and difficult decisions that have been at the core of medical decisions ever since healthcare professionals introduced artificial life supports (ventilators, dialysis, and resuscitation).

However, now we are seeing a new generation of medical breakthroughs creating new and ever more complex and difficult decisions to be made. Incredibly complex advances in biotechnology, pharmacology, immunotherapies, gene therapies, and life-altering and life-prolonging therapies are not solely about extending life; they inherently impact the quality of life during that extended period. Each new life-sustaining treatment brings further decision-making dilemmas to patients and their families.

How do patients and families emotionally and intellectually respond to the news that they can choose death or choose to undergo the newest *rescue* technology? As described by many who have made these choices, *it's a no-brainer*. Life is almost always chosen over death. The consequences of these decisions are hard to forecast and few want to let go of the promise of extended life. This contemporary dilemma is illuminated in the first illustrative case in this chapter. In addition to miraculous technologies to rescue patients from death, the growing expectations in our society contribute to unrealistic goals for medicine, often beyond reach.

Transarterial aortic valve repair in very elderly patients is becoming routine, implanted defibrillators and pacers have become ordinary, extracorporeal membrane oxygenation is offered for those who have profound heart and lung failure, and ventricular assist devices to support failure of heart function are just a few of the high-tech offerings for those who have irreversible organ failures. Experimental drug trials, risky surgeries, and stem cell transplantation for cancer and other diseases are offered as options when the only other option is to offer comfort medications and hospice. This forces patients and their families to choose between potential life extension or perhaps a better quality of life for a shorter period of time.

These and other complicated decisions driven by the armamentarium of treatment options available are compounded by the contextual issues surrounding each unique patient situation in our broader scope of society today. These issues include

1. financial burdens to cover the costs of life-prolonging interventions,
2. lack of caregiving supports for patients during extended illness and treatment,
3. choices for those who lack decisional capacity to articulate preferences,
4. vulnerable elderly patients who no longer have family as surrogate decision-makers,
5. undocumented patients with no payer source at all, and
6. familial discord and conflicting moral and religious beliefs about the *right thing to do*.

They all add to the overwhelming burdens placed on patients and family decision-makers to choose between life and death, and to understand the burdens versus the benefits of any given life-prolonging intervention.

Further complicating the milieu of decision-making in contemporary medicine is the frequent contrast between the medical provider's educated recommendation on the benefit of a particular intervention and the patient's or surrogate decision-maker's understanding of that benefit. Lack of trusting relationships with physicians and the healthcare system as a whole, religious and/or cultural beliefs and expectations, and coercive information ascertained through the internet and TV commercials all contribute to the conflicting opinions regarding options, choices, feasibilities, and expectations of medicine.

Bioethics consultants who practice in this current environment of acute care must be well-versed in traditional bioethical principles and mediation techniques, but must also be prepared and skilled enough to negotiate those cases that fall into the *liminal spaces* of moral uncertainty. The liminal space describes those circumstances in which we find little certainty about the moral acceptability of X and equal uncertainty about the possible harms of X.

The simple use of the four cornerstone principles is simply not enough to traverse the complex road of decision-making for seriously ill patients in contemporary medicine. The pressures of prolonging life pitted against the burdens placed upon the patient and the family to endure further suffering cause great anxiety and fears for families who believe they must make a decision that will prevent the death of a loved one or be *responsible* for that death.

Options are overwhelming in the face of uncertain prognostication. Many physicians are reluctant and poorly trained to give realistic prognoses when life is limited (Christakis 1999). The recent documentary *Being Mortal* (PBS 2015), by Dr. Atul Gawande, chronicles the excruciating task for doctors facing patients with honest, yet gentle, bad news. The burdens of high-tech and aggressive interventions are not fully understood until the outcome is experienced and then it may be too late to reverse the decision.

The devastating story of one patient in Dr. Gawande's documentary speaks to the heart of regret as her husband looks back at the burden of lost time getting more chemotherapy that could have been traded for better quality time with her family and new baby. These are the heartbreaking stories that highlight the difficulties of embracing today's medical *miracles* with enough information and reflection on your own goals to know which option to choose. Bioethics consultation can help when conflicting options are overwhelming in the face of serious illness.

This chapter is about the urgent need for the inclusion of bioethics in medicine. However, it would be remiss not to mention the invaluable contributions that palliative care medicine has made to help all patients with serious illness and their families. Palliative care is an added layer of care that can help in discerning the patient's goals of care and preferences that fit realistically with prognosis and treatment options. Palliative care interventions reduce suffering from pain and symptoms and improve the quality of life for countless patients and families. Palliative care differs from hospice care, providing simultaneously aggressive, disease-fighting treatments such as chemotherapy (www.getpalliativecare).

Traversing complicated ethical dilemmas to reach an end that is of greatest benefit to the patient according to her values and also nondestructive to the family and medical providers requires a higher level of training for hospital-based bioethics consultants than ever before. Certainly not every case of difficult decision-making requires the intervention of a bioethics consultation. However, when there is prognostic uncertainty, conflicting opinions, and significant burdens carried with treatment choices, bioethics should be at the table to support and help families, patients, and healthcare providers move toward the most beneficial resolution.

The clinical ethics consultants who step into the vortex of these difficult decisions among multiple stakeholders must have a solid depth of knowledge about the healthcare system with its competing incentives and driving forces. They should have an open relationship with providers, including a trust level to discuss expected outcomes honestly. Clinical ethics consultants must have an advanced knowledge and experience in ethical reasoning and analysis, excellent communication and mediation skills, and an intuitive sense of the array of emotions and fears that impact the patient, family, and stakeholders.

Discussions with patients and their loved ones require no less than these exquisite communication abilities along with extraordinary compassion and reflection in order to guide patients, families, and providers to a decision that is truly in the best interest of the patient and can be accepted as morally appropriate by the families and providers.

Most of the ethical dilemmas reviewed, retrospectively or prospectively, by bioethics committees in hospitals have been centered on end-of-life decision-making and, more specifically, the provision or withdrawing of artificial life supports. Issues regarding *futility* have emerged in contemporary medical ethics as the expectations among the public often exceed medicine's ability to restore functional life in those who are dying from their illness or injury. Unrealistic images of medical miracles promote this ethical dilemma, along with legal fears among physicians about refusing patient or surrogate demands for treatments they deem medically inappropriate or nonbeneficial.

There is national attention on recent recommendations for fair dispute resolution processes to address the increasing demands for scarce and costly resources for patients who will not benefit from an intervention and will likely not survive. The paradox in this country is the consistent demand for the individual freedom to *refuse* unwanted medical treatments, to attain a peaceful, comfortable death, even by means of physician aid in dying, and yet the equally consistent demand for treatments that are deemed by physicians to be medically inappropriate and nonbeneficial for the patient.

How do we reconcile the freedom to refuse with the demand to provide? Examples of such demands include feeding tubes for end-stage dementia patients, dialysis for patients who are in a permanent vegetative state, and resuscitation attempts for patients dying in the last stage of a terminal condition.

A formal academic background rich in ethical theories, principles, and history is certainly a prerequisite to entering the field of clinical ethics in a medical environment. However, it is not enough to venture into the abyss of clinical scenarios that rise to the level of needing ethical analysis and consultation. Beyond the academic background and understanding of ethical arguments, one must then acquire enough knowledge about the structure of medicine, the hierarchy of power within the institution, the unrelenting incentives that drive medical practice today, and how the environment of care and family dynamics affect the decisions that patients and their surrogates have to make in the worst of situations.

RECOMMENDED READINGS

American Society for Bioethics and Humanities (ASBH). 2011. *Core Competencies for Healthcare Ethics Consultation*, 2nd edition. The Report of the American Society for Bioethics and Humanities. Chicago, Illinois: American Society for Bioethics and Humanities.

Annas, G., and M. Grodin. 2016. "Second Thoughts: Hospital Ethics Committees, Consultants and Courts." *AMA Journal of Ethics* 18 (5).

Beauchamp, T. L., and J. F. Childress. 1989. *Principles of Biomedical Ethics*, 3rd edition. New York: Oxford University Press.

Charon, R. et al. 2017. *The Principles and Practice of Narrative Medicine*. New York: Oxford University Press.

Christakis, N. A. 1999. *Death Foretold: Prophecy and Prognosis in Medical Care*. Chicago University of Chicago Press.

Dubler, Nancy N., and Carol B. Liebman. 2004. *Bioethics Mediation: A Guide to Shaping Shared Solutions*. New York: United Hospital Fund of New York.

In re Quinlan, 70 NJ 10, 355 A2d 647 (1976).

Jonsen, A. R. 1998. *The Birth of Bioethics*. New York: Oxford University Press.

Kerwin, J. October 2007. *Impact of the Autonomy Model of Medical Decision-Making on Family Decision-Makers*. A doctoral dissertation for Caspersen School of Graduate Studies of Drew University, Madison, NJ. UMI Dissertation Services from ProQuest.

PBS. February 2015. "Being Mortal with Atul Gawande, MD." https://www.pbs.org/wgbh/frontline/film/being-mortal/. Accessed was April 23, 2019.

Tractenberg, P. L., ed. 2013. *Courting Justice: 10 New Jersey Cases That Shook the Nation*. New Brunswick, NJ: Rutgers University Press.

Chapter 2

A Model for Training Bioethics Consultants (for the In-House Seminar or Regional Workshop)

Jeanne Kerwin

This chapter models an instructional response to the call for the highest training of professionals serving as bioethical consultants within the American healthcare system.

In order to illustrate the complexity of contemporary ethical issues in medicine, participants in either an in-house seminar (extending over a negotiated number of meetings) or a regional workshop (occurring over a three-day conference) deliberate on several contemporary case studies. All of these cases are based on real-case scenarios, but the demographics have been changed to protect the privacy of the patient, family, and medical professionals.

The purpose of narrating and engaging in moral analyses of these cases is to illuminate the required ethical deliberation and reasoning, the need for mediation skills among disparate beliefs, and the requisite communication skills needed to clarify the issues and bring compromise and resolution for patients, their families, and the medical team.

Before presenting the cases for learning purposes, it is helpful to understand the steps that ethics consultants take when participating in consultations and the knowledge and skills that are required. The following steps are a general outline of the process but may differ given the unique circumstances of the case:

STEP ONE: IDENTIFY THE ETHICAL ISSUE

What is the reason for the consult request? What are the opposing views? Who thinks what and why?

It is important to discern ethical issues from other institutional issues that may give rise to an ethics consultation request. Frame the ethical question, for example, is it ethically appropriate to allow this forty-six-year-old woman in kidney failure to refuse dialysis based upon her belief that holistic therapies will improve her kidney function?

STEP TWO: GATHER ALL RELEVANT INFORMATION

Gather the relevant information needed for analysis of the case and the ethical question at hand; for example, the information related to the forty-six-year-old woman in kidney failure would include

The patient's current medical condition and history (from treating physicians/ medical record);
Prognosis with and without undergoing dialysis (from treating physicians);
Current treatments and life supports in place at time of consult;
The patient's cultural, religious, spiritual beliefs (from patient, family, others involved);
Information on holistic methods of treatment; and
The socioeconomic issues and other contextual issues (finance, caregiving, etc.).

STEP THREE: EXAMINE THE ETHICAL PRINCIPLES INVOLVED

Assess and respect the patient's autonomy:

Does the patient have decision-making capacity?
Does the patient understand options and consequent outcomes?
Has the patient expressed her preferences consistently?
Does the patient have a written Advance Directive?

Then consider the following:

Beneficence—What would be acting in her best interests?
Nonmaleficence—How should we prevent harm to the patient?

STEP FOUR: UNDERSTAND POSSIBLE LEGAL/POLICY ISSUES

Determine the following:

Hospital policy regarding withholding life-sustaining treatments,
Hospital consent policy, and

Advance Directives and Physicians Orders for Life-Sustaining Policies (POLST policies).

STEP FIVE: MEET WITH PATIENT, FAMILY, AND THE MEDICAL TEAM

Conducting a family meeting involves identifying key stakeholders to be present at the meeting and the following skills to run an effective ethics consultation meeting:

- Introductions and leveling of the playing field call for the art of active listening, facilitation skills that make sure all voices are heard and respected, and the practice of empathy and compassion that infuse the consultant's ability to articulate (frame and reframe) identified issues, mediate opposing views and emotions, build consensus, and summarize the key issues.
- When running a family meeting with a patient, family members, or friends of the patient, surrogates, and members of the medical team, it is important to begin by leveling the playing field. Family members are already overwhelmed with information and the complexities of the medical environment and may feel that this meeting is a "judgment" about decisions to be made. The field is not level to begin with because physicians and nurses with a high degree of medical knowledge are communicating with family members who, in general, are not knowledgeable about the field of medicine involving their loved one and are also emotionally entangled in the outcomes.

Leveling the playing field begins by the physical environment: meeting in a quiet place with chairs placed in a circle where everyone feels comfortable and included. Second, the consultant initiates introductions of those present and their relationship to the patient (e.g., I am Jane, the nurse taking care of your mother; I am Sam, the eldest son).

The ethics consultant should introduce the purpose of the meeting; following is an example introduction:

> We are convening at the request of your mother's medical attending to make sure that we all have the same information about her present clinical situation and prognosis; to find out more about your mother from you, her family who know her best, and to explore what might be her preferences if she were able to speak with us now. My role (as consultant) is to encourage an open dialogue about what you all feel is most important for her and to work towards a resolution within the guidelines of ethical principles, medical practice and her best

interests. Most importantly, as the bioethics consultant, I emphasize that the ethics consultant(s) will formulate an opinion and recommendations based upon our discussions, but clearly the decisions moving forward remain with you, as her surrogates and Dr. X., as her attending physician.

Opening the discussion should always be an invitation to each member of the family to have a chance to tell about their mother (a bit about her before she became ill), their understanding of her present illness, and what their expectations are after listening to her doctors. Most important family members express what they feel and think about what is most important at this point for her.

The invitation for discussion requires *active listening* by the ethics consultant with the requisite emotional support, validation of feelings, and respect and compassion (always have water and tissues on hand). Examples of listening actively are as follows: "I hear that you have cared for your mom for many years through her illness and coming to this point is very difficult for you"; "I recognize the frustration you are feeling with so many differing opinions coming from the various specialists treating her."

After the family/surrogates have ample time to speak from their perspective, a clear summary of the medical status and prognosis should be given (either by the physician in charge or by one who can relate the medical information). The family should then be encouraged to ask questions of the physician to make certain that they understand the information. Often the consultant will pause the medical summary to ask the physician to define the wording used or to explain a medical process that may be unclear to the family, for example, weaning from a ventilator versus withdrawing from the ventilator and why the withdrawing of artificial life supports when appropriate in terms of goals of care is not assisted suicide, euthanasia, and so forth.

Mediation and consensus building are essential dynamics in composing a summary of the issues on which bioethics consultant will build her recommendations. It is rare that an ethics consultation does not have some component of conflict, either among the family members or between the family and the medical team, as to what is the right action to take for the patient.

Mediation in bioethics is therefore a skill needed to reach resolution in most cases.

It is important to distinguish between mediation as a dynamic in the bioethics consultation and the consultation itself. Bioethics consultation is a substantive process in which the consultant gathers all of the factual information in the case. The consultant listens to the varying viewpoints and medical facts, and carefully explains the ethical principles involved (e.g., respect for autonomy, beneficence, nonmaleficence, justice, veracity) as well as any legal or policy constraints (such as aid in dying laws, doctrine of consent, advance directive law/policy). Ultimately, the bioethics consultant guides the stakeholders toward a principled resolution, one that is within the guide posts of ethical practice.

Mediation in bioethics is the use of accepted mediation techniques to identify, understand, and resolve conflicts among the parties. Mediation is more inclusive of the stakeholders and empowers them to articulate their position in a particular conflict, whereas bioethics consultation is more authoritative with regard to finding resolutions within the ethical framework. Mediation techniques are often employed within the bioethics consultation during the process.

Early bioethics consultants found in their practice that they needed to hone their mediation skills in order to accomplish resolution in cases of conflicting beliefs and understanding. Just opining about *the right thing to do* based upon the medical facts, the patient's known or unknown preferences, and the context of the case within ethics and the law was not enough to untangle the misunderstandings, emotions, and conflicts at the bedside of seriously ill patients.

Bioethics mediation differs from other mediation skills in many ways. The conflict is often about life and death. Time is usually of the essence. The mediator is also the bioethics consultant and needs to ensure that any resolution is not just a consensus among the stakeholders but is an outcome that is within ethical principles and within best medical practice guidelines. The patient is often not present and yet is the most important stakeholder at the center of the conflict. The mediator/consultant in bioethics is most often an employee of the hospital and the parties to the conflict do not sign an agreement to enter into mediation.

Examples of opening phrases in bioethics mediation follow:

> "Let me see if I understand what you are saying . . . . "
> "May I summarize what I believe you are both saying
> about the care of your mother . . . ?"
> "You are both saying that you love your mother and
> want what is best; and you, Bob . . . believe that . . . and Jane,
> you believe that . . . . "
> "I hear that you all love your mom but have differing
> thoughts on what she would think is best . . . let's
> hear each one of you . . . . "
> "Let's take a minute to reflect on why we are here . . . to
> focus on what your mom would want . . . . "

Reaching consensus is not the only goal of bioethics consultation and mediation. It is only the goal if the consensus also meets the best resolution within the ethical principles and best medical practices. For example, if a family reaches consensus that mother should have a Percutaneous

Endoscopic Gastronomy (PEG) tube for end-stage dementia, that is not within the best medical practices and violates the principle of beneficence and nonmaleficence for the patient (as artificial feeding tubes are not beneficial for end-stage dementia and are more burdensome/harmful than beneficial according to evidence-based medical practice).

Consensus building opens a space for all stakeholders to collaborate in resolving differences (perhaps in understanding or senses of directions or values that conflict) with the purpose of providing the care plan that benefits the patient within ethical principles and best medical practices. Consensus does not mean arriving at a unanimous decision or a majority vote. A consensus expresses the ability of all stakeholders to arrive at a sense of overwhelming agreement that even with some reservations the analysis and recommendations for the care of the patient reflect ethical principles and best medical practices.

STEP SIX: ETHICAL ANALYSIS

Ethical analysis includes examining all of the information from medical records, physicians, the patient, the family, and other stakeholders within the context of the relevant ethical principles, understanding the perspectives of the patient or surrogate, weighing and balancing the burdens versus the benefits of each option for the patient and formulating an ethical "opinion" about what resolution would be in the best interests of the patient.

STEP SEVEN: SUMMARIZE THE OUTCOME OF THE CONSULTATION

All ethics consultations should conclude with a written report to clarify and explain differing views, describing consensus achieved, if any, and the ethical opinion and recommendations of the consultation team. The patient and family should receive this information at the close of the meeting and the ethics consultants should advise the patient's medical team of the outcome, as well as entering the Consultation Report in the patient's medical record. This opinion is nonbinding and the decisions made remain with the patient or surrogate and the physician treating the patient.

With the consultative process set, participants now enter into bioethical narratives, case studies in which they imagine proceeding along the steps leading to a bioethics recommendation. When using case studies for consultation training, discussion of cases opens with the whole group contributing to a linear analysis and then proceeds into a role play of the case.

The narrative opens with the presentation of the facts of a case and then asks the students to

a. identify the ethical dilemma;
b. tell us what additional information they need to gather;
c. ask whom they would consider stakeholders to be involved; and
d. ask what the goals of a family meeting might be and their ethical analysis of the case.

Each case is unique and therefore elicits different questions. For example, if there is an unrepresented patient, the questions center on the ethical issue of who will make decisions and what the laws/policies might be that govern such in that setting.

When the learning strategy is a role play, the collaborative assigns one person to be the consultant and other participants play specific roles. For example, a participant may be assigned the role of a son who is a very religious person who has strong beliefs in miracles. There are no scripts per se, but the instructor provides a general written profile of who each person is and what their perspectives are about the case in point.

The consultant is not given a scripted role and is on *the hot seat* so to speak to run the meeting, seek the information needed from the stakeholders present, and make sure he or she hears from all the participants, mediates conflict, puts things in the ethical framework for analysis and context, and then summarizes his or her opinion/recommendation. In other words, the consultant would not know ahead of time that this son is very religious and believes in miracles. It would come out only if the consultant asks the son what he is feeling, thinking, and so forth. The instructor models the steps integral to consultative process.

It is difficult to describe role play exercises because each role play runs according to the content material of the case and has a learning life of its own. There are checks that an instructor puts in place, for instance, to interrupt the role play if it *runs off the rails* (following tangents); but role plays are extremely helpful for all participants; for example, people with differing moral or social horizons gain greater sympathy and understanding of one who has those strong beliefs, much like the religious son who believes in miracles.

Imagine now the linear or role play learning experience as you enter into each of the following case scenarios.

EXAMPLE CASE SCENARIOS

CASE 1: Fifty-eight-year-old male requesting to have his left ventricular assist device (LVAD) deactivated after thirteen months.

Hubbard has been a cross-country truck driver for the past thirty years, married with three children in their teens and early twenties. At the age of fifty-seven, he experienced sudden onset acute heart failure with unknown cause, possibly a virus. He was treated with conventional interventions and progressed to needing continuous home infusions of a medication to keep his failing heart functioning.

Eventually he was admitted to the hospital when the medication was no longer working. He was told that he needed either a heart transplant or a LVAD. He was shocked and terrified of needing a heart transplant and all of the aftercare and costs that a transplant might require. He chose to forgo trying to be approved for the transplant list and agreed to have the LVAD implanted as destination therapy. His wife and children all wanted him to get the LVAD so he could live. He felt he had to do this for his family but he was, not surprisingly, not very happy about the need to do this. He knew he could no longer drive a truck, and he wondered about his lifelong love of hunting, fishing, and swimming at the beach.

Hubbard agreed to the complicated open heart surgery required to install the LVAD into his chest and he and his wife were taught about the device and the maintenance it would require from them. They were shown how to keep the drive line coming out of his abdomen clean and dry, monitor the control device that showed the flow rate and other important measures, and how to maintain the batteries that he would carry on him in a vest-like garment.

Hubbard experienced multiple complications post surgery and had a long two-month stay in the hospital. Upon release he needed to spend another three months in a rehab facility to gain back his strength. When he finally returned home, his wife and he took over all the maintenance of the device with regular visits to the cardiac team. The stress on his family was significant. His wife had to work because he could no longer hold his job. They were financially in debt from the medical bills.

His children were upset at the disruption in their lives. Two of them were no longer able to attend college because of finances and were now working full time to help support the family. He could no longer participate in any of the activities that brought him joy: driving his truck, camping, hunting, boating, swimming, and playing softball in the local men's league. He also gave up Thursday nights with his buddies at the bar drinking beer and playing poker. He had progressively worsening fatigue and depression. His boys were depressed about losing the father they knew and loved.

Eight months after returning home and after several hospitalizations for complications, Hubbard made a request to the cardiac team to have the LVAD deactivated and have pain medications to accompany his death. He stated that his wife was about to file for divorce and described the extreme deterioration in his quality of life and the burdens that the LVAD was causing on all of them.

The cardiac team was understandably shocked by the request and advised Hubbard that they could not deactivate the device when it was working and keeping him alive. They felt that deactivating the LVAD would be "physician aid in suicide" and that Hubbard could live another five years with the LVAD and just needed more time to adjust to his new normal.

A bioethics consultation is requested to resolve the conflict between the patient's request and the medical teams' unwillingness to comply.

CASE 2: Thirty-seven-year-old female, twenty-four weeks pregnant, has large cerebral bleed leaving her in a coma. Neurology believes that she may progress to a permanent vegetative state and that a return of cognitive function is remote or impossible due to the extent of the brain injury. Her boyfriend (father of fetus) requests that she be removed from life supports and allowed to die. He states that his girlfriend did not want to be pregnant and he does not want to care for the child if it is born. They are estranged from any other family members and have been living in a nearby motel.

Bioethics consultation is requested, as the staff feel that the unborn child has rights and could survive if delivered by C-section and would have a better chance if they can keep the mother on the life supports for a few weeks more.

CASE 3: Forty-one-year-old quadriplegic from Motor Vehicle Accident (MVA) requests help in dying.

Joe is married, has no children, and was injured in a motorcycle accident nine months ago. His wife works as a waitress in the local diner at night but cares for him during the day, as they cannot afford any help at home other than the home health aid that comes under Medicaid benefit. He wants to stop eating and drinking in order to die but requests pain and symptom medications to help him achieve his goal.

Bioethics consultation is requested to discuss whether hospice can assist this patient in his quest to stop eating and drinking in order to die.

CASE 4: Eighty-nine-year-old female is admitted to hospital after suicide attempt and is now refusing intensive care treatment for respiratory failure.

Mrs. C. took a full bottle of Tylenol and a bottle of a sleep aids. She was brought to the hospital in a comatose state, treated in the intensive care unit (ICU) for the overdose, and placed on a ventilator for respiratory failure. She now has serious liver failure as well as respiratory failure and needs continued ventilator support for airway protection. She is awake enough to ask for the ventilator to be removed because she "wants to die." She has an Advance

Directive stating she never wanted any life supports to be initiated under any circumstances and she has a Do Not Resuscitate (DNR) order signed by her primary care physician.

Bioethics consultation is requested because the psychiatrist states that she is actively "suicidal" and therefore lacks decision-making capacity. He recommends that she be involuntarily committed to the psychiatric unit when medically stable. The ICU team has rescinded the DNR order and wants to keep her on the ventilator against her verbal request with the potential that she could recover. The son has arrived from out of state and requests that his mother's wishes to come off the ventilator be allowed and her wish to die naturally be honored.

CASE 5: An undocumented forty-two-year-old worker admitted with a large cerebral bleed leading to permanent vegetative state has been in the hospital for six months; he is now stable on tube feeding, dialysis, and full nursing care.

No nursing home will take him due to the fact that he has no payer source. He remains in a permanent vegetative state. His brothers insist that treatments continue and hospital staff not allow him to die. They await a miracle.

Bioethics consultation is requested because this patient has no money and no insurance. No nursing home will take him and the hospital cannot keep him indefinitely. He will never regain a cognitive, functional state, but his brothers insist that treatments continue to support him, as they believe a miracle will happen with American medicine and he will walk and talk again. They cannot provide financial support for him, nor can they care for him at home.

CASE 6: A sixty-one-year-old Down syndrome patient from a group home was admitted to the hospital twelve days ago with respiratory failure secondary to aspiration pneumonia and congestive heart failure.

He has a medical history of Alzheimer's disease diagnosed one year ago. He was intubated and put on mechanical ventilation in the ICU, where he has remained. The ICU doctors have recommended that he be withdrawn from the ventilator and placed on hospice comfort care with a DNR order, as they are unable to wean him from the ventilator and determine that his clinical decline cannot be reversed. The patient has a legal guardian for medical decisions appointed by the State Division of Developmental Disabilities.

A bioethics consultation is requested because the State Division of Developmental Disabilities (DDD) regulations mandate an ethics consult when there is any recommendation to withdraw life-sustaining treatments. The state-appointed guardian and a representative from Patient Rights NJ must be present at the consultation. The DDD regulations require a prognosis of life expectancy less than one year and a terminal diagnosis to allow the withdrawal of life-sustaining treatments.

These case scenarios illustrate the typically complex issues found in contemporary medical care that demonstrate the need for trained clinical ethics consultants to be available in hospitals, nursing homes, and, ideally, in all healthcare facilities. However, acute care hospitals have the greatest need to employ staff that can handle cases like these on a daily basis and often within an urgent time frame. Continued advances in medicine compel us to say *bioethics matters*, and we need qualified staff to attend to these patients, to their families, and to the providers who struggle to find the right options for treatment.

The general public is overwhelmingly unaware of modern medicine's abilities to extend life at all costs and the consequential outcomes that place families in untenable situations in which they must decide between continued life-supporting treatments and the death of the patient. The emotional burden of making such decisions can have lifelong repercussions on those family members.

Each case faced by ethics consultants is unique and requires information specific to that case. By following the steps described previously, for example, a case involving a young woman with a severe enduring eating disorder, who is refusing all attempts to provide her with nutrition, would require relevant information from experts about current treatment options and prognostic information on eating disorders.

A case involving vulnerable populations, such as the Down syndrome patient in case 6, would require knowledge about the state's regulations and process for ethical consultation for these patients. It is impossible to predict what issues may arise within the context of an ethics consultation. Sometimes family dynamics play a significant role in the ethical issue at hand; sometimes legal and policy questions confound the analysis; and sometimes the moral beliefs of the treating physician influence the conflicting views. Regardless, each case must be examined carefully for its own underpinnings, and the ethics consultant must recognize and reflect upon his or her own biases and beliefs to ensure they do not influence the resolution of the case.

RECOMMENDATIONS

There are formal training programs available throughout the United States, allowing hospitals to send a few selected staff to gain a basic education in bioethics. It must become a financial priority for senior leadership in healthcare to commit adequate funding and structure to create functional and accessible *bioethics committees*, with leadership that has education and expertise in all aspects of bioethics committee functions: policy review, education, and consultations.

After selecting leadership for the committee with academic background and expertise, creating an in-house *certification*, *designation*, or *authorization* process to have select members of the bioethics committee perform consultations is the second imperative for healthcare institutions. In-house training or the use of consultant trainers should include

1. developing a process for disseminating information and education about bioethics consultation services;
2. creating easy access to bioethics consultation throughout the institution for staff and patient families; and
3. developing a specific process of how consultations should be conducted, and, of key importance, standardizing the Bioethics Consultation Report format to be included in the patient's medical record upon completion of the consultation.

In addition, an evaluation process should be developed to monitor the successes, value, and/or opportunities for improvement in the services.

When bioethics committee members complete the training and have been mentored to the satisfaction of the bioethics leadership, they should be officially *certified*, *designated*, or *authorized* by the institution to perform bioethics consultations. This assures a level of expertise for handling the complex and emotional controversies that arise in the provision of modern medicine. An annual evaluation should be performed to reauthorize consultants based upon successful completion of consultations and continued education.

To provide the highest quality of bioethical analysis and conflict resolution, we cannot expect anything less than an assurance that our patients, their families, and our medical staff have access to a bioethics consultation service that provides educated and trained consultants with expertise and experience in this incredibly important role within all healthcare facilities.

INTERLUDE

Philip C. Scibilia

The shifts in medical practice from home and office to hospital and clinic exemplify the twenty-first-century redefinition of being a physician. Medical doctors have become members of teams treating patients in institutions governed by internal routines and external guidelines from government, insurers, and corporate owners (and, secondarily, religious authorities in some instances).

Increasingly, decisions are delegated to *bioethics committees*, which include nurses, lawyers, social workers, chaplains, philosophers, citizen representatives, patient advocates, and other people who are not physicians. Even if physicians dominate these care teams and hospital committees, their moral virtues or religious faith no longer confer moral authority. Any decisions must be articulate, defensible for both content and procedure and often, even in religious medical centers, by secular considerations. The next chapter illustrates a narrative approach to a specific issue that deepens insight into the complex ethical issues that healthcare providers face and enlivens ethics pedagogy.

Chapter 3

Drinking Stories: A Narrative Approach to Teaching the Neuroethics of Addiction

Katie Grogan

INTRODUCTION

Narratives and Neuroethics of Addiction is a one-hour workshop in which participants explore the ethical implications of the brain disease model of addiction (BDMA) through close reading and group discussion of a literary text. A narrative approach to this topic deepens insight into complex ethical issues and enlivens ethics pedagogy. Participants practice narrative scrutiny and apply this to the biomedicalization of addiction. Provocations about the BDMA are discussed. Suggested discussion prompts for workshop facilitation are provided.

This chapter describes the one-hour workshop, titled Narratives and Neuroethics of Addiction, in which internal medicine residents at one academic medical institution explore the neuroethics of addiction through a narrative lens. Workshop participants read and discuss "Big Blonde," a 1929 short story by Dorothy Parker set in Prohibition-Era New York, portraying the alcohol use disorder (AUD) of its main character, Hazel Morse.

Through literary analysis of the text and group discussion, participants consider the ethical implications of the biomedicalization of addiction. In particular, they contemplate the issue of volitional control that neuroethicists have long debated—if addiction is a disease that impairs autonomy, how much can we hold individuals experiencing addiction accountable for their actions?

Philosophical musings on the nature of free will and human behavior may seem frivolous in light of our current opioid crisis. Drug overdoses, primarily attributed to opioid use, now comprise the leading cause of death in Americans under fifty (Katz 2017a). The Centers for Disease Control (CDC) reports that more people die in this manner each year than are killed in motor vehicle accidents or by gun violence. The United States saw 70,237 drug overdose deaths in 2017, nearly 70 percent of which were opioid related. These deaths are increasing at an alarming rate, outpacing the HIV epidemic at its peak (Katz 2017b).

Substance use disorders (SUDs) comprise a public health emergency that incontrovertibly requires pragmatic medical, political, and social attention. Proposed responses, however, depend on how addiction is conceptualized, and how it is conceptualized depends on entrenched ethical norms and cultural values. A biomedical account of addiction as a disease of the brain is one model for conceptualizing this phenomenon.

Interrogating the norms and values that underpin this model is crucial to deciphering the story that it tells about addiction and understanding the implications of that story. This requires the skill of narrative scrutiny. The following discussion of the Narratives and Neuroethics of Addiction workshop offers instructional guidance for how to (1) utilize close reading of a literary text to practice narrative scrutiny and (2) use it to identify the risks and limitations of biomedical conceptualizations of addiction.

BIOMEDICALIZATION OF ADDICTION

The BDMA gained significant traction following a landmark 1997 report published in *Science* by Alan Leshner, then director of the National Institute on Drug Abuse (NIDA). He describes addiction as a chronic, relapsing disease of the brain, characterized by compulsive drug seeking and use.

The BDMA suggests that substance use is initially voluntary, but prolonged exposure can *hijack* the brain's reward system—a metaphorical switch is flipped, and the behavior is no longer a choice. The BDMA is supported, Leshner maintains, by observable differences in the structure and function of the addicted brain and the nonaddicted brain (Leshner 1997). During Leshner's tenure and that of the current director Nora Volkow, NIDA has pioneered groundbreaking research into the neurobiology of the BDMA and the precise mechanisms by which voluntary control becomes impaired (Volkow and Li 2004).

Current thinking suggests that addiction results from disruptions to the dopamine system. Addictive drugs cause the user to experience excessive dopamine increases. Constant exposure to these grossly distorted signals dysregulates the system. The user experiences decreased sensitivity to natural, physiological increases in dopamine (like food and sex), enhanced saliency value of the drug over other rational goals (like self-care or obeying the law), and poor inhibitory response (Hyman 2007; Volkow and Li 2004).

These changes, according to the BDMA, are responsible for the compulsive use and possibly the relapse patterns observed in individuals with SUDs.

These neurobiological insights have arguably uncovered "highly plausible mechanisms by which addicted individuals may 'lose control' over drug seeking and drug taking" (Hyman 2007, 10). That is to say, brain dysfunction impairs autonomy in persons experiencing SUDs.

The BDMA supersedes the outmoded moral model, which saw addiction as a matter of will, and condemned those experiencing it as weak or bad. Biomedical conceptualizations of addiction aim to offer not only a more evidence-based view of SUDs but also a more compassionate one. Indeed, neuroscientists often invoke destigmatization as a pragmatic defense of the BDMA: "The mere framework of BDMA has benefits in treatment as it significantly diminishes the stigma attached with addiction and gives hope for recovery to those fighting this devastating disease" (Volkow and Koob 2015, 678).

The promise of destigmatization hinges on how the BDMA figures volitional control: if the chronic use of addictive drugs alters the brain, ultimately undermining control and foreclosing choice, it is unreasonable to view the user as entirely blameworthy.

NARRATIVE DIMENSIONS OF THE BRAIN DISEASE MODEL

One might assume that the medical humanities, which has championed the imperative of empathy toward the ill, should endorse a framework like the BDMA that takes a benevolent stance toward addiction. However, attending closely to the narrative dimensions of the BDMA—subjecting it to careful narrative scrutiny—tells a more complex story and generates important ethical questions, including the following:

Are there risks of diminished control under the BDMA for autonomy more broadly?
Does too narrow a focus on the brain ignore other factors that contribute to addiction—like social context—to which research and resources ought to be directed?
How does stigma impact personhood, and do disease models truly mitigate stigma?

This chapter grapples with these questions by turning to a literary text and, in doing so, makes the case for a narrative approach to considering and teaching the neuroethics of addiction. What follows is an overview of the Narratives and Neuroethics of Addiction workshop, demonstrating how literature deepens insight into complex ethical issues and enlivens ethics pedagogy; it is not a detailed lesson plan. Suggested discussion prompts are indicated in italics.

Workshop participants are assigned "Big Blonde" in advance, along with one or two brief articles outlining the debate about volitional control under the BDMA. Steven Hyman's *The Neurobiology of Addiction: Implications for Voluntary Control of Behavior* and Neil Levy's *The Social: A Missing Term in the Debate over Addiction and Voluntary Control* work especially well (Hyman 2007; Levy 2007). The many other articles cited in this chapter comprise a suggested (though certainly not required or definitive) list of background readings as preparation for the workshop facilitator.

AGENCY AND ADDICTION

The workshop facilitator provides a brief introduction to the topic of neuroethics and addiction, emphasizing the issue of volitional control. The facilitator subsequently leads participants through a close reading. The ethical principle of autonomy is approached through its literary correlate, agency: the capacity of a character to act independently, make choices, or otherwise exercise control within the world of the story. A volunteer reads aloud an excerpt from "Big Blonde" in which the reader meets Hazel:

> She was a large, fair woman of the type that incites some men when they use the word "blonde" to click their tongues and wag their heads roguishly. She prided herself upon her small feet and suffered for her vanity, boxing them in snub-toed, high-heeled slippers of the shortest bearable size. The curious things about her were her hands, strange terminations to the flabby white arms splattered with pale tan spots—long, quivering hands with deep and convex nails. She should not have disfigured them with little jewels. [. . .] Men liked her, and she took it for granted that the liking of men was a desirable thing. Popularity seemed to her to be worth all the work that had to be put into its achievement. Men liked you because you were fun, and when they liked you they took you out, and there you were. So, and successfully, she was fun. She was a good sport. Men liked a good sport. (Parker 2003, 131–32)

Discussion is initiated through open-ended questions: *What do you notice?* More targeted questions help participants identify key narrative features, particularly the third-person narrator: *Who is telling this story?* The goal is not simply to acquaint participants with literary concepts like point of view and voice but rather to heighten participants' awareness of how these elements shape how this story (and every story) is told and their effect on the reader.

For instance, the third-person narrative mode situates Hazel in a framework that is out of her control. She is not permitted to tell her own story and is at the mercy of a disapproving narrator. This both reflects and amplifies the social context of the story—one in which others, namely men, set the rules. This point of view influences the way the reader sees Hazel. The narrator exclusively describes her in terms of her body and presents her imperfections—"flabby white arms splattered with pale tan spots"—as her most notable traits (Parker 2003, 131). She is introduced through the eyes of the men who appraise and critique her, an object for the consumption of others.

The reader is given no particularly compelling reason to like Hazel. The third-person narrative mode makes it more challenging to connect or identify with her than if she spoke the reader directly through a first-person account. She is positioned at a distance from the reader—a different "type," an "other"—thus, later in the story, as her AUD unfolds, she seems an even less relatable and sympathetic character.

Hazel's agency is compromised before her drinking even begins in that it is circumscribed by the normative gender dynamics of the time. Being a "good sport" may be a choice in so far as it requires deliberate actions on Hazel's part, but it is arguably her only choice, or one of only a few, for gaining economic stability and social mobility. Hazel's diminished agency is conveyed through various narrative features including the use of both passive language—"Her ideas, or, better, her acceptances, ran right along with those of the other substantially built blondes. [. . .] She summoned no alternatives"—and the passive voice—"She fell into the habit of going to Jimmy's alone. [. . .] The thought of death came and stayed with her" (Parker 2003, 132–44).

A nebulous timeline further emphasizes Hazel's insufficient agency. She is depicted as unable to properly manage or make use of her time: "She could not recall the definite day that she started drinking, herself. There was nothing separate about her days. Like drops upon a window-pane, they ran together and trickled away" (Parker 2003, 135). The temporal disorder of the narrative escalates as her AUD progresses: "More and more, her days lost their individuality. She never knew dates, nor was sure of the day of the week" (Parker 2003, 144).

Collectively, these elements contribute to the reader's sense of Hazel as a not fully agentic, autonomous character. This point is driven home in the imagery of the penultimate scene, which portrays Hazel as near-object, just barely a person, as she is subjected to inhumane treatment by a doctor.

Workshop participants discuss the difficulty of parsing what they can hold Hazel accountable for and what to blame on her circumstances. *Is Hazel responsible for her AUD? Are others responsible?* The conversation about her agency is used to problematize the concept of autonomy as it is traditionally taught and represented in the BDMA. The group explores possible limitations of the BDMA with respect to autonomy.

For instance, it assumes that individuals are equipped with roughly the same amount of autonomy. To be clear, the BDMA does account for genetic preloading, but it obscures the many external factors that impact the agency of certain groups and not others. This is an opportunity to acquaint participants with alternative models of autonomy often neglected in ethics pedagogy.

Unlike the dominant conceptualization of autonomy, which imagines self-sufficient agents making rational choices by exercising their innate free will, the feminist bioethical concept of relational autonomy contends that "agents are situated in historical, social, class, race and gender contexts," which mitigate their degree of autonomy (Stoljar 2011, 376). This can be done in a didactic manner or a dialectic one by asking questions that lead participants to discover relational autonomy: *Do all persons with capacity have autonomy? Do categorizations such as race, class, and gender impact autonomy?*

Additionally, the BDMA's emphasis on impaired autonomy presumably explains compulsive use and absolves individuals with SUDs of some degree of responsibility and moral judgment; however, impaired autonomy is precarious ethical territory, as it can be used to justify determinations about decisional capacity and impingements on liberty.

SOCIAL CONTEXT AND ADDICTION

Critics of the BDMA rightly assert that determinations about volitional control are not merely objective neurobiological findings; they are also culturally bound normative judgments. There is a strong tendency to view behavior that is deleterious to prized cultural values like autonomy as the product of a diseased mind (Foddy and Savulescu 2010). As ethicist Neil Levy explains, the BDMA "requires that we adopt an explicitly normative account of pathology, according to which someone suffers from a pathology when and only when they are subject to significant impairments of agency and consequently of the ability to pursue a good life" (Levy 2013, 5).

Such critiques do not dismiss the role of brain dysfunction in impaired autonomy all together, nor do they reinscribe the moral model of addiction; rather, they advise that too narrow a focus on the brain problematically views the individual in abstraction of her environment and obviates crucial social factors that play a causative role in her SUD. Levy's argument resituates the individual in her social context and recenters that context as a locus for inquiry in understanding and responding to addiction.

Workshop participants are asked to contemplate the environment in which Hazel is embedded: *How might you describe Hazel's social context?* As a woman in the 1920s, she is in a disenfranchised position, her choices severely limited by patriarchal social structures. Hazel is economically dependent on men and, following a divorce, she must secure a series of male suitors to support her.

Consequently, much of the story's action unfolds in heterosocial drinking situations—parties at her neighbor Mrs. Martin's apartment and dates with men at speakeasies—where Hazel's alcohol consumption is sanctioned and supervised by her male companions. Drinking is a requirement of being a "good sport"—a trope that pervades the narrative. The workshop facilitator encourages the group to unpack this concept: *What does it mean to be a "good sport" in this story? What does it involve?* On its face, "good sport" connotes an easygoingness but, paradoxically, closer reading suggests it demands vigilant self-control.

A volunteer reads aloud an excerpt:

> But she had to be careful of her moods with him. He insisted upon gaiety. He would not listen to admissions of aches or weariness. "Hey, listen," he would say, "I got worries of my own, and plenty. Nobody wants to hear other people's troubles, sweetie. What you got to do, you got to be a good sport and forget it. See? Well, slip us a little smile, then. That's my girl." [. . .] She was convincingly gay with him, though the effort shook her. "The best sport in the world," he would murmur deep in her neck. "The best sport in the world." (Parker 2003, 142–45)

Performing the *good sport* role is a tremendously effortful endeavor and the stakes are high. Hazel must contain and deny her own will to the satisfaction of her suitors in order to guarantee continuation of their arrangement, and ultimately her survival. Hazel's agency is depleted, as the confines of this role disallow her from exercising her autonomy. Her every move is so closely scrutinized by others, every misstep harshly admonished, that she must practice near-constant self-policing, especially around her emotions, as evidenced in the passage above.

Over the course of the story, Hazel experiences increasing dysphoria, as her need for self-expression is stymied by the role she must play. Subsequently, her alcohol use increases and her suicidal ideation begins. A volunteer reads aloud:

> She slept, aided by whisky, till deep into the afternoons, then lay abed, a bottle and glass at her hand, until it was time to dress and go out for dinner. She was beginning to feel toward alcohol a little puzzled distrust, as toward an old friend who has refused a simple favor. . . . She played voluptuously with the thought of cool, sleepy retreat. She had never been troubled by religious belief and no vision of an after-life intimidated her. She dreamed by day of never again putting on tight shoes, of never having to laugh and listen and admire, of never more being a good sport. Never. (Parker 2003, 144–45)

Workshop participants explore the correlation between these two factors—the debilitating effect of the incessant self-control intrinsic to the "good sport" role and Hazel's worsening AUD. Here, the facilitator introduces

Levy's use of the ego depletion paradigm in addiction. Derived from social psychology research, ego depletion suggests that self-control is a finite resource. When one is required to exercise self-control, it draws down one's reserve, ultimately exhausting it, thereby reducing one's ability to resist powerful urges. Ego depletion offers one model for how social context contributes to the behavior of individuals with SUDs—a factor often minimized under the BDMA.

A stressful or distressing environment can trigger ego depletion. If an individual with an SUD is immersed in an environment where she is bombarded with cues, she will experience persistent cravings that gradually deplete her self-control and make substance use inevitable. Conversely, if an individual is immersed in an environment where she rarely encounters cues, she may experience fewer addictive desires and, thus, less ego depletion.

An often-cited case example of the crucial role of social context in addiction and recovery is the relative success of Vietnam War veterans ceasing heroin use upon their return to the United States—a radically different setting than the one in which they became addicted (Levy 2007).

The facilitator prompts the group to identify the environmental cues in "Big Blonde": *Can we make the case for ego depletion in explaining Hazel Morse's AUD? Why or why not?* Participants may note the smallness of Hazel's world. She moves only between her apartment and various drinking establishments—settings saturated with alcohol-related cues. Moreover, the main characters in Hazel's life require that she drink in order to be likeable, making the environmental triggers inescapable.

Participants are then encouraged to reflect on ego depletion in their own patients: *Do you think ego depletion plays a role in the patients with SUDs whom you have treated? Does ego depletion impact the way you conceptualize or respond to these patients' illnesses?*

Focusing exclusively or primarily on the brain to uncover how chronic substance use impairs voluntary control misrepresents autonomy as a capacity originating solely from within the individual rather than one shaped heavily by environmental forces. Models that emphasize the role of social context may, in fact, more effectively destigmatize addiction than the BDMA because they diffuse accountability: "Blame should instead be shared: between the addict and the many social actors—from family, to the local, national and international authorities—that ensured that the addict would confront temptation, and which left the addict with weakened resources to cope with it" (Levy 2007, 36).

An overinvestment in the BDMA at the exclusion of social context also risks misallocation of resources, where funding for biomedical research and clinical treatments occludes population-level strategies to prevent addiction and reduce the social harms associated with it (Hall, Carter, and Forlini 2015).

STIGMA AND ADDICTION

To many scholars (social scientists in particular), the claim that disease models are beneficial because they are implicitly destigmatizing is deeply inaccurate. Not only are there innumerable examples of highly stigmatized diseases, both mental and physical, but there is also the question of whether the diseasing of a condition or behavior is itself stigmatizing. In the more than twenty years since its inception, the BDMA has failed to destigmatize addiction, stoking skepticism over the concept and whether its advocates really understand about how stigma works.

Stigma is often thought of as a negative judgment about a person or group of people due to a personal attribute or behavior that is perceived adversely in a given context. Put differently, stigma occurs when disapproval of what one does (for instance, use drugs compulsively) becomes disapproval of who one is (*a junkie*). In this view, stigma is a marker of anterior difference, meaning that social differences are seen as preceding the stigmas that they attract.

In contrast, researcher Suzanne Fraser and her colleagues characterize stigma as a performative process, meaning that stigma actually produces social differences, not the other way around. In this view, stigma "operates in the service of normative social relations," constituting certain identities as legitimate and credible and others as abject and discreditable (Fraser et al. 2017, 195).

Addiction comprises one such discreditable identity. But, as Fraser et al. explain, this is not because substance use constitutes inherently negative conduct but rather because society's normative understanding of autonomy creates the very conditions under which substance use emerges as a threat to free will. Stigma can render a person unintelligible to society, or *not quite human* (Fraser et al. 2017). Addiction stigma portrays individuals with SUDs as having diminished personhood on account of their impaired autonomy, and this has persisted despite the disease model.

The workshop facilitator briefly introduces these theoretical underpinnings and asks participants to reflect on Hazel's personhood: *In what ways is she portrayed as not quite human? Where do you see stigma at work in the story?* They may note the title and instances in which Hazel is simply referred to as *a blonde* or *big blonde*. She is metonymized to particular physical attributes: her blondeness, stereotypically associated with sexual promiscuity and unintelligence, and her body size. As a character, Hazel is meant to represent a general type rather than a specific individual.

Alcohol further dilutes her personhood:

The women at Jimmy's looked remarkably alike, and this was curious . . . the personnel of the group changed constantly. Yet always the newcomers resembled those whom they replaced. They were all big women and stout, broad of shoulder and abundantly breasted, with faces thickly clothed in soft, high-colored flesh. . . . They might have been thirty-six or forty-five or anywhere between. (Parker 2003, 141–42)

They are essentially proxies for one another. The tangential mention of Hazel's early employment as a model takes on greater significance: she is a literal stand-in, a prototype, but not the real thing, not a fully actualized and agentic person.

Stigma forces Hazel into an impossible double bind in which she must consume alcohol in order to be credible as a *good sport*, but drinking simultaneously makes her discreditable—it disqualifies her from being taken seriously and treated with respect by others. This mistreatment extends to the medical profession as well.

A volunteer reads aloud the scene in which a doctor arrives at Hazel Morse's apartment after she is found unresponsive. He initially believes she has drunk too much and callously tries to awaken her: "The doctor looked sharply at her, then plunged his thumbs into the lidded pits above her eyeballs and threw his weight upon them. [. . .] He flung her nightgown back and lifted the thick, white legs. . . . He pinched them repeatedly, with long, cruel nips, back of the knees" (Parker 2003, 150).

The doctor's insensitivity turns to ridicule when he learns she has taken an overdose of barbiturates in a suicide attempt: "He dropped Mrs. Morse's legs, and pushed them impatiently across the bed. 'What did she want to go taking that tripe for? Rotten yellow trick, that's what a thing like that is. Now we'll have to pump her out, and all that stuff. Nuisance, a thing like that is; that's what it amounts to. [. . .] You couldn't kill her with an ax'" (Parker 2003, 150–51). Hazel's substance use renders her "not quite human"—she is perceived as discreditable and unintelligible—and she is consequently treated inhumanely.

Workshop participants discuss how stigma shapes attitudes toward addiction in the medical community. That medical trainees subscribe to negative stereotypes about persons with SUDs is well-documented (Meltzer et al. 2013). *But does the BDMA alleviate this stigma? Might it actually reinscribe it?* Fraser and her colleagues contend that because stigma is part of a systemic process by which society organizes itself and categorizes subjects as legitimate or illegitimate (not merely a negative judgment of some fixed attribute or behavior), calling addiction a disease is unlikely to successfully destigmatize it.

In fact, some evidence suggests that the BDMA "entrenches stigma by rendering people both sick and therefore not competent to 'speak back' against this rendering" (Fraser et al. 2017, 199). In Fraser's own study, interviewees reported that the connotations of illness and suffering that come with the diseasing of addiction do not resolve stigma. The notion that individuals with SUDs should not be stigmatized for their drug consumption because addiction is a disease that impairs autonomy ignores the fact that diminished autonomy itself, whether by disease or otherwise, carries stigma in a culture that profoundly values free will and the rational, choosing subject.

In a 2014 interview study, researcher Stephanie Bell and her colleagues found that while most neuroscientists and clinicians believe that the BDMA is beneficial to persons experiencing addiction, others believe it can have adverse effects. The disease model can foster learned helplessness, diminish motivation to seek help, and undermine the belief that one can change one's own behavior. Interviewees used phrases like "permanent condition," "done deal," and "my brain's f**ked" (Bell et al. 2014).

The message that individuals with SUDs are sick, and their substance use is caused by a brain disease for which they are not responsible, suggests an anterior difference. It is a biological one, not a moral one, but an anterior difference nonetheless—the very thing to which stigma attaches itself. Conceptualizing addiction as a disease that impairs free will may, instead of lifting the stigma and humanizing addiction, risk further marginalizing and impinging on the liberty of those afflicted.

For instance, the BDMA, on the premise of insufficient autonomy, could be used to condone paternalistic medical practices and coercive treatment (Berghmans et al. 2009). As Fraser et al. warn, "Measures that treat stigma as a fundamentally individual phenomenon . . . not only ignore its institutional dimension, but actively obscure and naturalise it, potentially ushering in abuses of power" (Fraser et al. 2017, 197).

Hazel Morse is certainly a case example of the interplay between diminished agency, substance use, stigma, and paternalism. Her plea at the end of the story, "Why couldn't he let me alone?" in reference to the doctor who revives her, though indicative of the severity of Hazel's mental distress and suicidality, is a poignant request by a woman who wants powerful others to stop controlling her will (Parker 2003, 151).

REPLICATING THE WORKSHOP

This chapter and the workshop it describes are not intended to impugn the BDMA or suggest that addiction is not best understood as a disease of the brain. Rather, the preceding discussion has sought to demonstrate that the biomedicalization of addiction does not mark unmitigated progress. Though it offers tremendous neuroscientific insights into SUDs, the BDMA also carries significant ethical implications that are deserving of close attention, especially by those involved in the provision of patient care.

In the context of medical education, learners should be encouraged to scrutinize the BDMA in order to discern the story about addiction that it tells. Like any story, it originates from a particular point of view and is steeped in particular norms and values. For this reason, studying a literary text, such as Parker's "Big Blonde," is an ideal exercise for practicing such narrative scrutiny.

If one were interested in replicating the Narratives and Neuroethics of Addiction workshop at one's own institution, it is recommended that two facilitators with different training colead it, as addiction is a topic that engages multiple disciplines. For instance, the author has partnered with addiction psychiatrists, philosophers, and medical historians. Each collaboration shapes the workshop into slightly different iterations, but all inevitably lead to rich cross-disciplinary dialogue and bioethical insights about the vastly complex issue of addiction. Though this workshop is taught to residents, it can be easily adapted for learners across the medical education spectrum.

REFERENCES

Bell, Stephanie, Adrian Carter, Rebecca Mathews, Coral Gartner, Jayne Lucke, and Wayne Hall. 2014. "Views of Addiction Neuroscientists and Clinicians on the Clinical Impact of a 'Brain Disease Model of Addiction.'" *Neuroethics* 7 (1): 19–27. https://doi.org/10.1007/s12152-013-9177-9.

Berghmans, Ron, Johan de Jong, Aad Tibben, and Guido de Wert. 2009. "On the Biomedicalization of Alcoholism." *Theoretical Medicine and Bioethics* 30 (4): 311–21. https://doi.org/10.1007/s11017-009-9103-7.

Foddy, Bennett, and Julian Savulescu. 2010. "A Liberal Account of Addiction." *Philosophy, Psychiatry, & Psychology : PPP* 17 (1): 1–22. https://doi.org/10.1353/ppp.0.0282.

Fraser, Suzanne, Kiran Pienaar, Ella Dilkes-Frayne, David Moore, Renata Kokanovic, Carla Treloar, and Adrian Dunlop. 2017. "Addiction Stigma and the Biopolitics of Liberal Modernity: A Qualitative Analysis." *International Journal of Drug Policy* 44: 192–201. https://doi.org/https://doi.org/10.1016/j.drugpo.2017.02.005.

Hall, Wayne, Adrian Carter, and Cynthia Forlini. 2015. "The Brain Disease Model of Addiction: Is It Supported by the Evidence and Has It Delivered on Its Promises?" *The Lancet Psychiatry* 2 (1): 105–10. https://doi.org/10.1016/S2215-0366(14)00126-6.

Hyman, Steven E. 2007. "The Neurobiology of Addiction: Implications for Voluntary Control of Behavior." *American Journal of Bioethics* 7 (1): 8–11. http://search.ebscohost.com/login.aspx?direct=true&db=rzh&AN=106192509&site=ehost-live.

Katz, Josh. 2017a. "Drug Deaths in America Are Rising Faster Than Ever." *New York Times*, June 5. https://www.nytimes.com/interactive/2017/06/05/upshot/opioid-epidemic-drug-overdose-deaths-are-rising-faster-than-ever.html.

Katz, Josh. 2017b. "Short Answers to Hard Questions about the Opioid Crisis." *New York Times*, August 10. https://www.nytimes.com/interactive/2017/08/03/upshot/opioid-drug-overdose-epidemic.html.

Leshner, Alan I. 1997. "Addiction Is a Brain Disease, and It Matters." *Science* 278 (5335): 45 LP-47. https://doi.org/10.1126/science.278.5335.45.

Levy, Neil. 2007. "The Social: A Missing Term in the Debate over Addiction and Voluntary Control." *American Journal of Bioethics* 7 (1): 35–36. http://search.ebscohost.com/login.aspx?direct=true&db=rzh&AN=106192521&site=ehost-live.

Levy, Neil. 2013. "Addiction Is Not a Brain Disease (and It Matters)." *Frontiers in Psychiatry* 4 (April): 24. https://doi.org/10.3389/fpsyt.2013.00024.

Meltzer, Ellen C., Alexandra Suppes, Sam Burns, Andrew Shuman, Alex Orfanos, Christopher V Sturiano, Pamela Charney, and Joseph J. Fins. 2013. "Stigmatization of Substance Use Disorders among Internal Medicine Residents." *Substance Abuse* 34 (4): 356–62. https://doi.org/10.1080/08897077.2013.815143.

Parker, Dorothy. 2003. "Big Blonde." In *Under the Influence: The Literature of Addiction*, edited by Rebecca Shannonhouse, 131–52. New York: Modern Library.

Stoljar, Natalie. 2011. "Informed Consent and Relational Conceptions of Autonomy." *Journal of Medicine and Philosophy* 36 (4): 375–84. https://doi.org/10.1093/jmp/jhr029.

Volkow, N. D., and George Koob. 2015. "Brain Disease Model of Addiction: Why Is It So Controversial?" *The Lancet Psychiatry* 2 (8): 677–79. https://doi.org/10.1016/S2215-0366(15)00236-9.

Volkow, N. D., and Ting-Kai Li. 2004. "Science and Society: Drug Addiction: The Neurobiology of Behaviour Gone Awry." *Nature Reviews Neuroscience* 5 (12): 963–70. http://10.0.4.14/nrn1539.

INTERLUDE

Philip C. Scibilia, DHM

Ethics has expanded well beyond the Hippocratic Oath tradition of medical ethics that was focused on the responsibilities of the individual practitioner for his or her patient. The issues now encompass the ethical implications of a broad variety of health-related decisions, including not only decisions affecting individuals but also the effects of societal actions in the health field: issues of a social justice nature. This past chapter addressed addiction; the next addresses the ethics of racial equity.

Chapter 4

Calling for Racial Equity Training in Medical School Curriculum

Kirk Johnson

Historical and social competency about race is an important quality doctors need to adequately interact with and diagnose minority patients. Unfortunately, racial equity training is a scarce resource in medical schools. Consequently, implicit bias and microaggressions are realities that compromise nonmaleficence between minority patients and doctors. The next two chapters provide an overview of the usage of race equity in U.S. medical school curriculums and offer an instructional model, Race Talk workshops, as an initial pedagogical step toward race equity implementation in medical education.

INTRODUCTION

It is no secret that communities of color have faced a host of challenging health issues. In fact, numerous studies have shown the ways minorities suffer from health inequities in the United States. In American medicine, "epidemiological data has reflected and reinforced scientific thinking about race for more than 200 years" (Graylee, 48). Epidemiological data show an overwhelming amount of evidence of racial inequalities in morbidity and mortality, which African Americans rank the highest. For example, the age-adjusted death rate for African Americans was 30 percent higher than whites.

Specifically, rates from hypertension, kidney disease, diabetes, hypertensive renal disease, and septicemia are twice as high in African Americans as in white Americans. With respect to heart-related issues in particular, "cardiovascular disease accounts for the largest share of black-white difference in mortality (34.0%), but there are substantial contributions from infections (21.1%), trauma (10.7%), diabetes (8.5%), renal disease (4.0%), and cancer (3.4%)" (Graylee, 48).

Such horrible statistics are a result of a historical disregard of African Americans by the American medical system. For example, the discrimination behind the Tuskegee, Henrietta Lacks, and other similar studies are disturbing historical events that demonstrate ways in which African Americans have become victims of a medical system that has placed discriminatory labels and racial markers. Racial discrimination is the unjust treatment, consideration, and distinction of a certain race because of personal characteristics associated with race.

Racism is the belief that all members of each race possess characteristics or abilities specific to that race, especially to distinguish it as inferior or superior to another race or races. Labels enforced on minority patients produce negative assumptions and preconceived notions by the doctor. The consequence of labeling is a huge mental strain on minority patients. This is an important factor in communities of color. Negative factors that contribute to poor mental health outcomes include "unfair treatment and social disadvantage as well as other social stressors, such as inadequate levels of social support, neuroticism, the occurrence of life events, and chronic role strain" (Mays et al. 2007, 206).

Labels also create poor communication, which in turn worsens health disparities. A patient having a transparent relationship with their physician is more likely to have better health outcomes. In contrast, a patient feeling judged is more reluctant to discuss their health because they feel condemned by a false label attributed to them, which worsens personal and collective health outcomes. Therefore, it is imperative that doctors have the proper education, historical competence, and interpersonal training regarding race as a significant factor in the social determinants of health for communities of color.

An effective way to accomplish important attributes is for medical schools to have mandatory courses and training focused on racial equity. According to the Center for Assessment and Policy Development, racial equity is the condition that would be achieved if one's racial identity no longer predicted, in a statistical sense, how one fares.

Racial equity is one part of racial justice and includes work to address the root causes of inequities not just their manifestation. The elimination of root causes encompasses policies, practices, attitudes, and cultural messages that reinforce differential outcomes along the lines of race or failure to eliminate them. However, there are many challenges that stand in the way of making racial equity training a reality. A primary challenge is overcoming the lack of inclusion and diversity.

INCLUSION AND DIVERSITY

The term "diversity" has been used a lot, but it doesn't solve the problem of creating affirming environments that value and welcome people of color. It is important to acknowledge that our American education history had social consequences of exclusion and segregation of students of color. Our American medical education history is no exception. The racist structures of this history, like mass incarceration, gentrification, the achievement gap, racially selective admissions, and many more obstacles, haven't gone away in communities of color.

Medical education needs sustained inclusion and diversity. Diversity asserts that one is different, which can be interpreted as being abnormal, unusual, or *the other*. Inclusion embraces one's differences and lived experiences. It asserts contribution and effective perspectives. Inclusion emphasizes belonging.

The lack of inclusion in medical schools presents a huge setback in inclusive and diverse education. For medical schools to be culturally and socially effective, its administration, faculty, staff, and students should reflect the general population. It is evident that "African Americans, Hispanics, and Native Americans compose only 12.3% of the nation's physician's workforce despite representing 37% of the US population" (Maldonado 2014, 605). Based on these statistics, it makes sense that curriculum dealing with racial equity is rare, because the individuals making curriculum-based decisions, most of the time, are not from communities of color.

As a result, racial competency and learning development remain stagnant. Studies have shown that inviting doctors of color to participate in career days, academic support, mentoring, loan repayment programs, and scholarship information sessions has diversified many medical departments and programs (Maldonado 2014, 606). As a matter of fact, Boston University School of Medicine has an *Early Medical School Selection Program,* which offers mentorship and summer medical classes to black, Latino, and Native American students. More medical schools should incorporate similar programs to have a racially balanced student roster.

In order to foster progress, inclusion is necessary in the admissions and hiring process. Medical education should embrace pioneers like Dr. Daniel Hale Williams and Dr. Thomas C. Unthank.

In 1891, Dr. Williams founded the Chicago's Provident Hospital and Nurse Training School (Gamble 1995, 11). It was the first black-controlled hospital. Black hospitals treated African Americans with respect and dignity. In other hospitals, race mattered more than class in the quality of care a patient received. The fear of medical experimentation, death, discrimination, and mistrust embolden blacks to want their own hospitals.

African Americans experienced value and compassion interacting with doctors who understood black life in American society. Williams made a national declaration for black-owned hospitals. Williams' decree did not only involve hospitals to care for the sick but also a means for medical education for black doctors and nurses who had very few options to practice medicine. Kansas City General Hospital No. 2, also known as KC Colored Hospital, was the first major hospital for black patients with white staff.

Dr. Thomas C. Unthank founded two small private hospitals: Douglass Hospital in Kansas City, Kansas, in 1898 and Lange Hospital in Kansas City, Missouri, in 1903 (Gamble 1995, 9). In 1914, Kansas City General was the first hospital to be managed by an African American when Dr. William J. Thompson became the superintendent and Mary K. Hampton-Brown named superintendent of nurses. Ten years later, all departments had black leadership.

Other black-controlled hospitals included Tuskegee Institute and Nurse Training School in Alabama stabled in 1892; Fredrick Douglass Memorial Hospital and Training School in Philadelphia, established in 1895; and Home Infirmary Clarksville, Tennessee, established in 1906 (Gamble 1995, 11). In 1912, 63 black-controlled hospitals existed, and by 1919 almost, doubled to 118 (Gamble 1995, 3).

Throughout the twentieth century, black hospitals have closed due to financial strains and buyouts. There are only two black hospitals left. However, due to conflicting sources and hospital closures, it is hard to give an accurate number of black-owned hospitals in 2019. I gathered two hospitals from reliable sources. The Chicago Provident Hospital known as Provident Hospital of Cook County was taken over by the Cook County Bureau of Health Services and Howard University Hospital in Washington, D.C. (Gamble 1995, 194–95).

Due to the work of Dr. Williams and others, there is a positive outlook today that "healthcare professionals from underrepresented groups are more likely to work in medically underserved areas, and race concordance in patient-physician relationships result in higher patient satisfaction and trust in the health system" (Maldonado 2014, 605). The idea *to take care of your own* still permeates.

There are indicators of a preferential turn to racial-ethnic, cultural, and gender diversity among medical residents of color. "Residency candidates from underrepresented groups place strong emphasis on the ethnic diversity of the city, patients, house staff, and faculty and are interested in an academic environment that supports ethnic minorities" (Maldonado 2014, 606). Diverse experiences and interactions are deciding factors not only for students and residents of color but also for students in general. About one-fourth of seniors in American medical schools reported that cultural, racial-ethnic, and gender diversity is a *highly important factor* in their residency program decision (Maldonado 2014, 606).

Cross-cultural experiences and relationships enrich medical residents personal and professional development. An efficient pedagogical means for medical students before residency is a comprehensive curriculum that incorporates critical race theory (CRT).

RACE THEORY

According to the *Oxford Research Encyclopedia*, CRT is a framework that offers researchers, practitioners, and policymakers a race-conscious approach to understanding educational inequality and structural racism to find solutions that lead to greater justice. In a medical lens, CRT has connection to health disparities. In a 2017 survey, 92 percent of U.S. Family Medicine department chairs reported their medical school curriculum included aspects of racial and ethnic disparities (Chen et al. 2017, 1–3).

Many department chairs were not satisfied with course quality and content in their programs. There was not any quantitative and qualitative measurement to accurately measure the quality and effectiveness of curricula. Similar surveys suggest a disconnect about physician's knowledge about race, human genetics, epigenetics, and the causes of health disparities (Bolnick 2015, 362).

Health disparities are important to incorporate in curricula, but such inquiry only focuses on the symptom not the source. What needs to be examined is the concept of race itself, and how it has shaped our social institutions, social systems, which leads to the consequence of health disparities. This is the work of racial equity in medical education.

Studies have shown that

> there is nothing in the medical curriculum like the critical race theory that has flourished in legal studies since the late 1980s when some law schools, with more elective time and a long tradition of incorporating critical social theory and history into coursework, began integrating critical race theory into their curricula. (Braun 2017, 521)

Solidifying the importance of humanities and social sciences, the U.S. Medical Licensing Exam and Medical College Admission Test (MCAT) integrated sections in national exams. Medical humanities complements racial pedagogy in medical school curricula. Medical school faculty unfortunately do not have the competency to adequately teach CRT.

A medical humanities program gives medical schools the opportunity to hire scholars that specialize in complexities of race and medicine. Also, medical humanities introduces faculty and students to other areas that complement CRT like history of medicine, medical anthropology, research ethics, bioethics, medical narrative, palliative care, and other medical humanities-based courses. In addition, medical humanities is a tool for medical schools to reconsider its pedagogy and usage of race, which is not a biological reality but a social and political construction.

American influences of self-identification came from Carl von Linnaeus and Johann Fredrich Blumenbach. Swedish botanist Carl von Linnaeus (1707–1778), known as the *father of taxonomy*, created the classification of skin color and first modern study of man. German anthropologist Johann Fredrich Blumenbach (1752–1840) included skin color, skull, and the physiognomy of man in five categories and coined the term "Caucasian" from the Caucasus mountains (Bethencourt 2014, 250–53). Linnaeus and Blumenbach are important figures in the classification of racial groups.

Since 1950, the United Nations Educational, Scientific and Cultural Organization (UNESCO), the American Association of Physical Anthropologists, the International Union of Anthropological and Ethnological Sciences, the American Sociological Association, and the American Anthropological Association all agreed that race is not a proxy for biological explanations and difference (Bliss 2012, 3). Yet the concept of race as an explanation for disease is still infiltrating science and medicine in the twenty-first century.

The previously named institutions have indeed contributed to great progress on how we should view race in science and medicine. However, their bold statements do not erase the ingrained societal effects of racial ideologies in American society. The precedent of racial self-identification was never set by individuals, but by the U.S. government over such individuals. The U.S. Office of Management and Budget (OMB) constructed racial and ethnic categories used to collect, organize, and analyze the country's demographic data. OMB changed racial categories at least ten times since its inception in 1800 (Wailoo et al. 2012, 52). For example, the first U.S. Census listed

> Free White Male, Free White Female, Other Free Person, and Slave. During the nineteenth century, additional categories that fell in and out of use included Free Colored Person, Black, Mulatto, Quadroon, Octoroon, Indian, Chinese, and Japanese. The twentieth century saw a new proliferation of categories including Hindu, Korean, and Negro. (Kahn 2013, 28)

On May 12, 1977, the OMB's Statistical Policy Directive No. 15, Race and Ethnic Standards for Federal Statistics and Administrative Reporting was produced to provide

> standard classifications for record keeping, collection, and presentation of data on race and ethnicity in Federal program administrative reporting and statistical activities. These classifications should not be interpreted as being scientific or anthropological in nature, nor should they be viewed as determinants of eligibility for participation in any Federal program. They have been developed in response to needs expressed by both the executive branch and the Congress to

provide for the collection and use of compatible, nonduplicated, exchangeable racial and ethnic data by Federal agencies. (CDC 1977)

After many changes, this process of taxonomy (classification) led to the categories of race and ethnicity we know today: American Indian or Alaska Native, Asian, black or African American, Native Hawaiian or Other Pacific Islander, with Hispanic or Latino and Not Hispanic or Latino as the two categories for ethnicity (Kahn 2013, 28). The OMB's categories are used on the local, state, and federal levels for research, data, and practice, which are used for public health issues and biomedical research.

The U.S. Patent and Trademark Office (PTO) has powerful influence through federal officials controlling the use of race into biomedicine. The PTO's decisions produce constructed racial categories used for the U.S. Census. The racial categories are used as a means of biological research that supports the appropriation of race and biology in biomedicine. In fact, genetic research has rapidly grown since the completion of the Human Genome Project (HGP) in 2003.

The HGP was an international research effort to sequence and map all the genes of humanity, also known as the genome. The mass amount of data and knowledge obtained was tremendous. Such knowledge needs to be collected, stored, and classified as genetic information. The OMB and PTO racial categories are used in international biobanks. Hence, international federal governments sponsored data banks to maintain genetic data for biomedical researchers.

These data banks and databases are the National Institute of General Medical Sciences under the Department of Coriell Human Genetic Variation Collections, the DNA Polymorphism Discovery Resource (PDR), the database of single-nucleotide polymorphisms (dbSNP database), the Haplotype Map Project (IHMP or HapMap), the National Center for Biotechnology Information (NCBI or GenBank), the DNA DataBank of Japan, and the European Molecular Biology Laboratory (Kahn 2013, 30).

These databases have unprecedented power in determining how genetic information is used. Researchers use these databases to organize racial categories and genetic information and apply genetic data by race classification. For example, the PDR's chief scientists, who were from the HGP, created race-based sample sets by federal race classification (Bell and Figert 2015, 179).

Biobanks romanticized race with biomedicalization using classification. Classification is the assignment of organisms to groups within a system of categories distinguished by structure and origin. It implies class, order, and phylum (race, stock, or kind) of individuals and groups. Additionally, classification is defined by ethical choices that hold meaning and enable identification.

However, classification inevitably excludes an individual or group as *the other* allowing different forms of hierarchy. Genetic classification profoundly describes the essence and character of a human being down to the cellular level. Genetic classification demonstrates power and danger because "it involves biological categories that may be confused and conflated with race. Any resulting reification of social categories of race as biological constructs risks new forms of exclusion and stigma" (Kahn 2013, 33). Regardless of the disunion between race and biology, harmful ideas of race continue to reify in medical education.

In 2016, two first-year medical students of color expressed concern regarding their textbook illustrating that *normal* gums are bright and pink (Gowda et al. 2017, 274). Also, the criterion for a newborn baby's health is its pink appearance. Recent studies in dermatology suggest that black Americans with melanoma, a type of skin cancer, are more than four times as likely as white Americans to be diagnosed only after their cancer has already spread to other parts of the body (Cormier et al. 2006, 1907–14). Half of dermatologists report that their medical schools did not prepare them to diagnose cancer on black skin (Buster et al. 2012, 53–59).

In addition, barely one in ten dermatology residencies include a rotation in which physicians-in-training gain specific experience treating patients with skin of color (Nijhawan et al. 2008, 615–18). Such ideas of skin color and the lack of people of color represented in medical textbooks assert white supremacy, which is the belief that individuals who are categorized as *white* are inherently superior and have inherent value compared to people from other racial groups.

Such assertions are troubling and are consequences of an American medical racial history that has not been reconciled. Today, eugenics is condemned. Ironically, however, ideas of race that were shaped by eugenic thinking still exist in normal science, even in the use of "licensing examinations [that] perpetuate racial stereotypes, albeit unintentionally" (Braun 2017, 254). Consequently, unwarranted ideas of race are difficult to retract. The same goes for physicians' perceptions of race.

Many physicians believe that there are genetic differences between races, which explain racial health disparities (Bolnick 2015, 362). It is apparent that the concept of race is engrained within our culture and society. Medical education has a responsibility to correct the pedagogy, research, and ideologies that assert race and biology have correlation. This is an immense task, but it is achievable.

If medical education does not deal with perceptions and usage of race directly, health and social inequity will continue to remain. In making racial equity-focused pedagogy and continuing education, racial equity workshops as requirements are helpful in developing racial competency and solidarity among physicians.

REFERENCES

Bell, Susan E., and Anne E. Figert. 2015. *Reimagining (Bio)Medicalization, Pharmaceuticals and Genetics: Old Critiques and New Engagements.* New York: Routledge.

Bethencourt, Francisco. 2014. *Racisms: From the Crusades to the Twentieth Century.* Princeton, NJ: Princeton University Press.

Bliss, Catherine. 2012. *Race Decoded: The Genomic Fight for Social Justice.* Stanford, California, CA: Stanford University Press.

Bolnick, Deborah A. 2015. "Combating Racial Health Disparities through Medical Education: The Need for Anthropological and Genetic Perspectives in Medical Training." *Human Biology* 87 (4), 361–371.

Braun, Lundy. 2017. "Theorizing Race and Racism: Preliminary Reflections on the Medical Curriculum." *American Journal of Law & Medicine* 43 (2/3). https://journalofethics.ama-assn.org/article/avoiding-racial-essentialism-medical-science-curricula/2017-06.

Braun, Lundy, and Barry Saunders. 2017. "Avoiding Racial Essentialism in Medical Science Curricula." *AMA Journal of Ethics* 19 (6).

Brooks, Katherine C. 2015. "A Silent Curriculum." *JAMA: Journal of the American Medical Association* 313 (19), 1909–1910.

Buster, Kesha J., Erica I. Stevens, and Craig A. Elmets. 2012. "Dermatologic Health Disparities." *Dermatologic Clinics* 30 (1).

CDC. 1977. "Statistical Policy Directive No. 15, Race and Ethnic Standards for Federal Statistics and Administrative Reporting." CDC, May 12. http://wonder.cdc.gov/wonder/help/populations/bridged-race/directive15.html.

Chen, Frederick, Frederica Overstreet, Allison Cole, Amanda Kost, and Joedrecka Brown Speights. 2017. "Racial and Ethnic Health Disparities Curricula in US Medical Schools: A CERA Study." *PRiMER* 1. https://journals.stfm.org/primer/2017/chen-0010

Cormier, Janice N., Yan Xing, Meichun Ding, Jeffrey E. Lee, Paul F. Mansfield, Jeffrey E. Gershenwald, Merrick I. Ross, and Xianglin L. Du. 2006. "Ethnic Differences among Patients with Cutaneous Melanoma." *Archives of Internal Medicine* 166 (17), 1907–1914.

Gamble, Vanessa Northington. 1995. *Making a Place for Ourselves: The Black Hospital Movement, 1920–1945.* New York: Oxford University Press.

Good, Mary-Jo. 2013. "Culture, Race, and Hierarchy." *Culture, Medicine & Psychiatry* 37 (2), 390–397.

Gowda, Deepthiman, Laura J. Benoit, and Christopher I. Travis. 2017. "A Common Purpose: Reducing Bias in the Curriculum." *Academic Medicine* 92 (3).

Gravlee, Clarence C. 2009. "How Race Becomes Biology: Embodiment of Social Inequality." American *Journal of Physical Anthropology* 139 (1), 47–57.

Kahn, Jonathan. 2013. *Race in a Bottle: The Story of BiDil and Racialized Medicine in a Post-Genomic Age.* New York: Columbia University Press.

Maldonado, Maria E., 2014. "The Role That Graduate Medical Education Must Play in Ensuring Health Equity and Eliminating Health Care Disparities." *Annals of the*

American Thoracic Society 11 (4). https://www.atsjournals.org/doi/full/10.1513/AnnalsATS.201402-068PS

Mays, Vickie M., et al. January 2007. "Race, Race-Based Discrimination, and Health Outcomes among African Americans." *Annual Review of Psychology* 58.

Nijhawan, Rajiv I., Sharon E. Jacob, and Heather Woolery-Lloyd. 2008. "Skin of Color Education in Dermatology Residency Programs: Does Residency Training Reflect the Changing Demographics of the United States?" *Journal of the American Academy of Dermatology* 59 (4), 615–618.

Roberts, Jane H., Tom Sanders, and Val Wass. 2008. "Students' Perceptions of Race, Ethnicity and Culture at Two UK Medical Schools: A Qualitative Study." *Medical Education* 42 (1), 45–52.

Wailoo, Keith, Alondra Nelson, and Catherine Lee. 2012. *Genetics and the Unsettled Past: The Collision of DNA, Race, and History*. New Brunswick, NJ: Rutgers University Press.

Chapter 5

Racial Equity: A Pedagogical Model

Kirk Johnson

The instructional model in this chapter responds to the call for race equity training in medical school education. The pedagogical praxis addresses in either a dialogical seminar or an extended workshop format the unconfessed dynamics that have led to resistance to the educational transformation needed when regarding race and healthcare education.

The caveat concerning talking about race is vulnerability. Currently, there are no models to defuse tension between doctors discussing race and privilege (Good 2013, 392). White doctors talking about race have a tendency to become uncomfortable, emotional, and fearful. Feelings of guilt, denial, defensiveness, sadness, and frustration are described as *white fragility*. *White fragility* is known as the defensiveness and avoidance that arise for white people when facing even a minimum amount of racial stress.

An example of *white fragility* in a medical school setting was in a qualitative study done in two United Kingdom (UK) medical schools. The results of the study mentioned white students being fearful discussing race-related issues, medical students of color being viewed as different, and barriers to talking about race (Roberts et al. 2008, 45–52). In addition, such feelings were evaluated by medical resident Katherine C. Brooks' article in the *Journal of American Medical Association*. Brooks asserts,

> But regardless of intent, the message I got was clear. I've learned to minimize the pain, forgo the consent, blame the behaviors, and dismiss the concerns of my patients of color. I've witnessed missed opportunities for healing and the loss of patient trust. And I believe that if we refuse to deeply examine and challenge how racism and implicit bias affect our clinical practice, we will continue to contribute to health inequalities in a way that will remain unaddressed in our curriculum and unchallenged by future generations of physicians (Brooks 2015, 1909–10).

These are normal reactions discussing race. Such emotions and feelings need to be expressed, examined, and resolved in a space, culture, and mission that embraces dialogue without fear of consequences. Pedagogical approaches using emotional intelligence should be incorporated in medical school curricula. Deep racial examination in the clinical practice starts with recognizing one's biases, which is self-awareness.

A pioneer in the field, Dr. Daniel Goleman emphasizes the basic tenets of emotional intelligence: self-awareness, awareness of others, and awareness of one's surroundings. Though emotional intelligence wasn't exclusively developed for doctors regarding race dialogue and interaction, it is a necessary practice. Incorporating emotional intelligence in dialogues and curricula on race is a helpful aid in overcoming the barrier of *white fragility* in racial discussions.

Racial awareness is done by students applying and articulating the principles of bioethics, which are beneficence (doing good), nonmaleficence (do no harm), autonomy (freedom), and justice (equity) in nonreligious and religious settings, as these are applied to racial problems in medical and healthcare practices. The process of dissecting those ethical principles draws connections between the medical-ethical issues regarding race equity, the history that has shaped current society, and the students' personal and professional development through engaged pedagogy. Engaged pedagogical practices allow medical students to be active, responsible, and accountable. *Race Talk Workshops* are an effective teaching and training method for racial equity.

PRECONDITIONS FOR RACE TALK WORKSHOPS

Race Talk Workshops allow racial dialogue about experiences between students of color and white students. To start, workshops should have two facilitators to lead the group. Using a two-facilitator model avoids pressure on one facilitator to lead a group on a weighted topic like race. Both facilitators can benefit from each other's strengths and understanding about racial dialogue through training.

Facilitators should be trained in race dialogue and history before offering *Race Talk Workshops*. There are many credible organizations that provide opportunities for training like the *American Council on Diversity, OpenSource Leadership Strategies, The People's Institute for Survival and Beyond*, and *Race Forward*. Anti-racism organizations vary on their approaches. All medical institutions are different and should carefully review what type of training for *Race Talk Workshop* facilitators would be effective in their culture.

Facilitators do not have to be experts on race. Their role is to guide conversations about race, monitor conversation time, and balance workshop time. Facilitators should not exude an unrealistic and condescending *savior mentality* that asserts saving everyone from their biases, prejudices, and systematic racism. They should have a passion for racial equity, be open-minded, careful listeners, nonjudgmental, understand body language, and be able to effectively handle emotions and tensions that naturally come with racial dialogue. In addition, facilitators should ask questions and clarify comments when appropriate.

Since most medical schools' student population are white, it is suggested facilitators should be white for three reasons. First, medical students of color (and people of color in general) have voiced their experiences about racism for centuries. There is a profound solidarity when white individuals speak against racism, a topic that does not negatively affect white facilitators' livelihood. Second, it alleviates the burden of a facilitator, who is a person of color, *representing and speaking on behalf of an entire race*: An experience many people of color have when trying to express their lived experiences in an environment that is dominantly white. Third, the facilitation by a trained white individual alleviates cognitive dissonance.

A minority facilitator can be misunderstood as complaining or being irrational due to cognitive dissonance of white students. However, if a white facilitator acknowledges difficult experiences only people of color encounter, it can hold more resonance to white individuals. These elements have a positive impact on *Race Talk Workshop* group dynamics.

Including facilitators, *Race Talk Workshops* should have eight to ten individuals per group. Workshops should meet once a week for fourteen weeks. The time frame should be two hours and ten minutes with a ten-minute break in between. Workshops should be in a private, quiet, and intimate setting so that participants can feel comfortable in talking, showing emotion, and sharing personal information.

It is essential that the curriculum leadership develop with the facilitators a Race Workshop Curriculum drawn from the experiences of students, faculty, staff, and administration—the institutional race-related issues. The development of that curriculum opens an avenue for the creation of a *Race Talk Covenant* for facilitators and students to follow. Confidentiality, respect for others, and listening to others should be core principles of the covenant. Facilitators and workshop participants agree and comply with the covenant. It is rare that a covenant gets broken. However, if that happens, the medical institution should have a disciplinary process in place. Finally, the workshop group demographics should be as diverse as possible, given the social limitations of medical school student communities, including different races, sex, gender, and sexual orientation to provide different lived experiences and perspectives.

THE RACE TALK WORKSHOP: AN INSTRUCTIONAL NARRATIVE

Led by facilitators, workshops should start with a *mindfulness* exercise called the relaxation response for five minutes. Individuals sit comfortably in a circle. Facilitators guide participants through a mindful setting aside of all distractions. There is a seven-step process:

First, pick a word or phrase that is an important to racial equity (i.e., solidarity, unity, humility, awareness, etc.).
Second, sit quietly in a comfortable position.
Third, close your eyes.
Fourth, relax your muscles.
Fifth, breathe slowly and naturally, repeating the focus word or phrase selected softly to oneself as one exhales.
Six, assume a positive attitude, listen for, look for what prompts a calming spirit of gratefulness in your spirit.
Seven, continue steps one through six for five minutes.

After the *mindfulness* exercise, facilitators should do an icebreaker connected to the outlined topic for the workshop. The first workshop session should allow participants to introduce themselves as part of the icebreaker exercise. Perhaps, each participant might recognize with the group one's focus word or phrase and what they became mindful of as the exercise progressed. Workshop participants can *pass* if they are not ready to speak right away, but should respond once ready to share. This method is particularly useful if the participant is emotionally uncomfortable and behaviorally agitated.

If the participant needs to step out of the room, then he/she should be allowed to do so. Being able to *pass* gives the participant time to constructively process their emotion and behavior. In addition, facilitators should politely intervene if one participant is dominating the conversation. A great response would ask other workshop participants a question, what they think about the previous comment, or to share a relevant story. Facilitators should remind participants to speak from personal experiences and use *I* statements. Generalities are not useful.

Facilitators will go over their medical school's approved *Race Talk Workshop* curriculum. *Race Talk Workshop* curriculum should be structured based on the current issues of the institution. For other workshop sessions, a case study, news article, short videos, documentaries, or a journal article can be great icebreakers and workshop activities. However, based on the facilitators' discretion, other means can be used for icebreakers. Depending on the medical institution's discretion, workshops can have a set curriculum for the fourteen weeks or facilitators can ask participants at the first workshop what race-related topics they want to discuss.

A suggested fourteen-week workshop curriculum includes the following:

Week 1: White Privilege
Week 2: Racial Representation in Society
Week 3: Colorblindness/Light versus Dark
Week 4: Implicit Bias
Week 5: Microaggressions
Week 6: Distinctions among Stereotypes, Prejudice, and Discrimination
Week 7: Dynamics of Race in Space/Place
Week 8: White Fragility
Week 9: Structural Racism
Week 10: Economics of Race
Week 11: Race and Education
Week 12: Criminal Justice
Week 13: Race as a Biological Myth
Week 14: Health Disparities

In Week 1, the workshop group talks about *white privilege*, which is a term for the way people and social institutions grant social privileges that benefit white people beyond what is commonly experienced by people of color under the same social, political, or economic circumstances. *White privilege* is not something that white people necessarily do, create, or enjoy on purpose. It refers more to the phenomenon that social systems award preference based on the presumptions of white as norm. In Week 2, the group will explore the social dynamics of *whiteness* or white people being the norm in society compared to people of color who are considered abnormal.

In Week 3, the group examines the notion of *colorblindness*. *Colorblindness* is the act of denying or refusing to acknowledge that people's race and people's lived experience in America because of their race differs. This is reflected in statements like, *I don't see race, I'm colorblind, I don't see color, We are all equal,* and *But we're all just one human race.* Also, the group will reflect on the meanings and feelings behind light and dark.

In Week 4, the group observes *implicit bias*, which takes the form of unconscious attitudes, stereotypes, and unintentional actions (positive or negative) toward members of a group merely because of their membership in that group. These associations develop over the course of a lifetime through exposure to direct and indirect messages. When people are acting out of their *implicit bias,* they are not even aware that their actions are biased. In fact, those biases may be in direct conflict with a person's explicit beliefs and values. The preference for associating with people like oneself racially in a class or professional gathering, or the tendency to allow preconceived attitudes toward a person of color that might influence an employment decision—for example, the association of a name that sounds black or brown.

In Week 5, the group deliberates on *microaggressions*. *Microaggressions* are the result of *implicit bias*, wherein a statement, an action, or an incident is indirectly or subtly (often unconsciously) reflective of prejudice. An example would be a person clutching their bag as they walk by a black man. In Week 6, the group clarifies the distinctions among *stereotypes*, *prejudice*, and *discrimination*. A *stereotype* is an oversimplified generalization about a person or group of people without regard for individual differences. *Positive stereotypes* that link a person or group to a specific positive trait can have negative consequences.

Prejudice is the prejudging or deciding about a person or group of people without enough knowledge. Prejudicial thinking is frequently based on stereotypes. An example of prejudice is pain treatment toward patients of color. In *The New York Times*, an articletitled *Minorities Get Less Pain Treatment in E.R.* highlighted a study by the Centers for Disease Control and Prevention (CDC), which concluded white patients receive more pain treatment in emergency rooms than African Americans and other minorities do. As discussed, *discrimination* is the denial of justice and fair treatment by both individuals and institutions in many areas, including employment, education, housing, banking, and political rights. Discrimination is an action that can follow prejudicial thinking.

In Week 7, the group uncovers the dynamics of race in space and place. People of color, specifically Hispanics and blacks, are under constant social surveillance under the suspicion they are doing something wrong. In Week 8, the group reflects on *white fragility*, mentioned previously; it is bias described as the defensiveness and avoidance that arise for white people when facing even a minimum amount of racial stress. The feelings can be so uncomfortable that white people distance themselves from engaging or actively shut down conversations about race. It may surface as the outward display of emotions, such as anger, fear, and guilt, and behaviors such as argumentation, silence, and leaving the stress-inducing situation.

In Week 9, the group discusses *structural racism*. As previously described, Power + Prejudice = Racism. Racism describes the result of prejudicial attitudes being combined with the power to dominate and control the systems and institutions capable of carrying out discriminatory practices. Racism results from access to the power that enforces prejudices to advantage one racial group.

In Week 10, the group reflects on the consequences and connections between race and economics. Weeks 11 and 12 deepen the conversation about the social consequences of race. During Week 11, the group explores the challenges communities of color experience in the education system. In Week 12, the group discusses how notions of race are deeply rooted in the criminal justice system. In Week 13, the group examines race as a biological myth and how that myth should change ideas, treatment, and research. Lastly, in Week 14, the group discusses health disparities and how the topics of the previous thirteen weeks are connected to health disparities and the social determinants of health.

Race Talk Workshops should be a constructive space to reflect on workshop sessions and topics. Each workshop should focus on the assigned or proposed topic. Side conversations are distracting and should not be permitted. Participants should journal at least once a week about the group's conversations, being mindful of their emotions, thoughts, insights, and responses to the conversations (using the same exercise that opens the workshop to attend to what one's mind, heart, and spirit are saying). Furthermore, participants can evaluate how bioethical principles were followed or broken through shared stories or experiences in the workshop.

The effective way for participants to take stock of what they have learned, their awareness of self and society, especially the medical community, regarding race and equity opens a reflection on their journals. The workshop experience of mindfulness regarding race stirs participants' moral imaginations—seeing what the next instructional step would be in preparing students for medical practice informed by racial equity. That reflection would provide the substance of an ensuing conversation between members of the workshop in which they imagine and design collaboratively a proposal for the medical school's curriculum leadership.

The objectives of the workshops invite participants to demonstrate analytical and critical thinking skills regarding race and equity in conversations and in writing, and to successfully interact with other participants and facilitators sharing what they become mindful of—the ideas, stories, emotions and personal, as well as social ethical judgments.

Workshop outcomes help participants become aware of the connections between race, power, and privilege, their manifestations and consequences. When we are honest about how race has functioned and continues to be perpetuated, there can be dialogue about how to address its causes and the necessary reconciliation and redistribution of power and opportunity. As race is a difficult topic, participants will demonstrate competent oral communication skills as a result of engaging in workshops by considering multiple perspectives when discussing lived experiences. As a result, knowledge and skills for living in a diverse society are developed or strengthened. *Race Talk Workshops* are a promising intervention. Despite the challenges of inclusion and diversity in curricula, some progress has been made.

CONCLUSION

The Society of Internal Medicine's Health Disparities Task Force, the American Medical Association Foundation, the Academic Alliance for Internal Medicine, the Association of American Medical Colleges, and the Association of Schools of Public Health all claim to have curricula that deal with health disparities and cultural competence training for doctors (Maldonado 2014, 605). The Accreditation Council on Graduate Medical Education (ACGME) has the Clinical Learning Environment Review (CLER). CLER's goal is to "identify how sponsoring institutions engage residents in the use of data to improve systems of care, reduce health care disparities, and improve patient outcomes" (Maldonado 2014, 604). These interventions have been established within the last six years.

The University of California San Francisco's School of Medicine launched a new curriculum accompanied by diversity training in 2016. The Brown University and the Warren Alpert Medical School have an initiative called *Pathways to Diversity and Inclusion*. The University of New Mexico School of Medicine, Albert Einstein College of Medicine, Columbia University College of Physicians and Surgeons, and the Mayo Clinic of College of Medicine have programs dealing with race, medicine, and health. Mount Sinai School of Medicine has a critical theory and activism elective. Also, Dartmouth School of Medicine has a social justice curriculum (Braun 2017, 254). All these interventions have been established within the past three years.

In 2013, the Alliance of Academic Internal Medicine (AAIM) changed the name the Association of Professors of Medicine to the AAIM Diversity and Inclusion Committee. The committee's purpose is to support women and people of color in academic medicine to promote diversity and inclusion in residency programs as well as medical schools and departments of medicine (Maldonado 2014, 606). These interventions set an optimistic tone that medical organizations and schools are trying to create more training and awareness on race and its complexities in medicine. However, creating safe spaces to dialogue about race is crucial in the effectiveness of curricula and training.

Focusing exclusively on health disparities is therefore only evaluating half of a bigger problem in communities of color. Prioritizing race equity–focused pedagogy and continuing education models like workshops for physicians is a suggested approach. In addition, when physicians strengthen their emotional intelligence, transformation occurs, and the work of racial equity can effectively begin.

REFERENCES

Braun, Lundy. 2017. "Theorizing Race and Racism: Preliminary Reflections on the Medical Curriculum." *American Journal of Law & Medicine* 43 (2/3), pp. 239–256.

Brooks, Katherine C. 2015. "A Silent Curriculum." *JAMA: Journal of the American Medical Association* 313 (19), pp. 1909–1910.

Good, Mary-Jo. 2013. "Culture, Race, and Hierarchy." *Culture, Medicine & Psychiatry* 37 (2).

Maldonado, Maria E., 2014. "The Role That Graduate Medical Education Must Play in Ensuring Health Equity and Eliminating Health Care Disparities." *Annals of the American Thoracic Society* 11 (4).

Roberts, Jane H., Tom Sanders, and Val Wass. 2008. "Students' Perceptions of Race, Ethnicity and Culture at Two UK Medical Schools: A Qualitative Study." *Medical Education* 42 (1).

INTERLUDE

Philip C. Scibilia

As the United States becomes more diverse, there will be increased need to establish the validity and reliability of constructs and instruments across racial, ethnic, and cultural groups. Researchers need to continue to examine how ethnic differences in risk aversion and patient preferences influence medical decision-making and health outcomes. In addition, perceived discrimination, racial bias, and stereotyping should be legitimate healthcare education questions. More education is needed to influence these factors significantly, contribute to the resolution of healthcare disparities, and identify and put into practice strategies to eliminate their effects on health. There is little precedent in our medical-ethical tradition for determining the way in which these important social contributions should be considered in defining medical responsibility and in resolving such questions as what care should be available to which segments of the population.

The final two chapters offer a model for healthcare education rooted in an ethics of equity—a practice that the voice of the vulnerable, the pain sufferer, informs, and transforms. Professor Kopchinsky's contributions combine the social-ethical analysis of the specific clinical issue of pain management.

Chapter 6

Hearing the Voice of the Sufferer: The Moral Compass of the Healthcare Professional

Gaetana Kopchinsky

> Although concealed in a blanket of unbearable suffering, the essence of our humanity lies within the resilience of our unique and everlasting spirit.

This chapter is an inquiry into the complex construction that defines and characterizes the human experience of pain. Instructors find their way through the management and semantics of pain in stories told by people in pain. Those stories prompt the much-needed design and implementation of a medical humanities seminar on pain for healthcare professionals, especially physicians.

INTRODUCTION

The exploration of pain is a journey of *invisible epidemic* proportions (Morris 1991, 57). There are distinct conceptualizations that physicians and scientists, past and present, have considered and still explore in terms of the correlation between the causation and the amelioration of pain. The dilemma of pain management has become a distinct specialty.

The powerful, dynamic story of pain (its etiology and unique expressions as told by scientific discoveries and cultural biases) is a relational construction. The narrative begs communication with others for relief and comfort while at the same time craving some kind of safety from its isolation and despair. And so the experiences of pain sufferers search for a voice. Who speaks for those in pain?

BACKGROUND

Pain is perhaps the oldest affliction known to humankind. Its conception has been defined through the lens of psychology, literature, science, and certainly religion. Through the ages, the idea of suffering has shared a general comparison to pain. Religious and philosophical narratives provide metaphors and stories regarding pain, for example, the biblical accounts of those who have endured pain and suffering as a test of their commitment to and faith in both society and a higher being. Moral philosophers have even measured pleasure versus pain as a definition of worth in terms of social values.

To that point, historically, the reality of suffering has raised many doubts for many religious followers in terms of the absence of humanity. The first question becomes, Why is there suffering at all? Is it something human beings deserve? Is it something capricious that simply strikes all of us, good and bad alike? Alternately, does suffering have any point, or purpose? If we think of pain as deserved, should we seek a reason [for this particular suffering]? (Lammers and Verhey 1987, 248). Lammers and Verhey propose a theory of human isolation and despair as pain sufferers' only companions.

As far back as scribes could record the vestiges and meaning of oral history, pain has been labeled a medical problem—even a disease. Persistent pain becomes a top reason people seek medical care, yet current solutions fall short or sometimes have unendurable side effects. The good news is recently neurobiologists have identified a number of cellular and molecular processes that lead to the initiation and maintenance of pain (Stuckey et al. 2001, 11845–846).

THE PHILOSOPHICAL DILEMMA

According to Plato, "The medical art is good, and it is for the sake of health [and well-being] that medical art is good, is it not?" (Pellegrino 2001a, 559).

In terms of the amelioration of pain, there is a dilemma due to the social construction of consensus and dialogue surrounding the idioms of experienced pain. Therefore, has a normative morality anchored the external practice of medical ethics in treating pain? If yes, should this creation become the essence and nature of the clinical encounter between physicians who treat the symptoms of a patient with seemingly unmeasurable suffering?

Plato, Aristotle, and later in the thirteenth century Thomas Aquinas in somewhat related fashion treated the welfare of humans as the *telos* of human activity. In other words, *What is the purpose of this life?* In resolving the ends and good of human life, in terms of everyday existence, the ends and the means *to the good* are intimately intertwined. There have been discussions and debates from the late thirteenth and fourteenth centuries to our contemporary times as to the foundations of a teleological ethic, but that foundation has been seriously eroded.

Is there a rupture between ethics and physiology? Is there an insistence on locating the good in the will and ethics in reasoning about internal pain/suffering alone? Is there any logical connection between fact and value? Hume's denial of any connection between *is and ought, fact and value* and his preference for affect over reason in ethics as well as G. E. Moore's declaration that the good is an indefinable quality lead us to an ultimate dilemma: is there any moral resolve to eliminating pain in its entirety, or not (Pellegrino 2001, 567)?

There is a skeptical view of certain aspects of *good* ethics in terms of human behavior, particularly in the relief of pain. In an effort to illuminate a traditional approach to relieving pain, contemporary philosophers seek a holistic attitude in looking at the mental, physical, and emotional elements of its construct:

> The kind of dialogue that would be most productive is not nostalgic immersion in the past but recognition of a cultural heritage that belongs to all humans, and is stored in a perennial philosophy constantly renewed and revitalized, but not eradicated by new thought. (Pellegrino 2001b, 672)

> In view of the ethical component to doing [good] for the sake of a truthful acknowledgment of the brokenness of the world, we must therefore face and acknowledge the pain of another with humility, and see suffering, honestly. (Lammers and Verhey 1987, 247)

THE ROLE OF A PHYSICIAN WITHIN A SOCIAL CONTEXT

According to historian M. Pernick (1985), the role of the European physician was one that both sought to relieve pain, in an effort to service the patient through use of opium and laudanum, and inflict pain to relieve the spread of infection, and much more. This strange relationship between relief and infliction follows society throughout the ages. It may even be observed that the physician valued pain as a sign of the patient's vitality, and as a measurement of the prescription's effectiveness.

It is the contemporary job of the medical humanist to analyze where we are today in terms of a human response to pain sufferers. As Thomas Merton has told us, What is really new is what was here all the time. This really new is that which may every moment spring freshly into existence (quoted in Pellegrino 2001b, 672). And so, in spite of adversity, it is important for healthcare professionals to examine the hopeful legacy of a tradition of ethics in terms of pain and the longtime suffering our society experiences and as cultures and as social contexts evolve (Pellegrino 2001a).

MORTAL ILLS BECOME ACTS OF HEROISM IN OUR STORIES

A medical practitioner needs special introspective skills and courage to appreciate a patient's profound transition from suffering to peace. Clinicians are not specially equipped to deal with abstract human conditions. Richard B. Gunderman, physician and author, reflecting on the early days of his medical training, recounts a relationship with a patient suffering from a rare form of bone cancer.

He recalls the following:

> In the hospital, it was the habit [of this patient] to roam the halls late at night after his wife and small children had gone to their lodging. I never asked him whether it was pain that kept him moving or perhaps loneliness and a simple desire for conversation. One night, having completed my work for the day, feeling too tired to read on my own, and facing no other prospect but to give in to sleep, I felt like talking. On that night, and on other nights following, we discussed nothing in particular. Our conversation might turn to his aspirations at work . . . or to my thoughts about medicine. For a time, he would talk about his plans for the future as though they were still foremost in his mind, but before long he would lapse into the past tense and grow sullen. I think that a part of him was looking for encouragement, but what I knew of his condition made medical reassurance nearly impossible. I hid from his pain by focusing on the bright side of things. It was a kind of dishonesty; though at that early point in my medical training I did not recognize it as such. One night, after I had been away for several days, I met him again in the semi-dark hallway near the nurses' station. He was asking a nurse to bring something to his room. . . . For some reason, she proceeded to introduce the two of us—a rare event by possible standards. Equally strange, neither he nor I spoke up to say that we already knew one another. I put out my hand to shake his, and he started to do the same; then it hit me. His arm was missing. It had been amputated as part to his treatment. I should have anticipated the amputation . . . but it came as a surprise to me. In the instant before my hand withdrew and I looked down, at a loss for what to say or do, I caught in his eyes a look of sorrow, perhaps even shame. I begged his pardon, but we did not speak further . . . we never met again and I regret not knowing him better to this day. (Gunderman 1990, 15)

A week or so later, the patient died, and the physician was disturbed that nothing in his medical training or the principles of medical ethics had prepared him for or guided him to attend to the man's silent pain and suffering.

Such stories show that the most well-meaning clinician needs a commitment, a multifactor desire, to consider the personal nature of pain and suffering. That dedication reaches beyond physiological treatment. There is evidence that many independent medical clinicians and humanists, such as Richard Gunderman, Benjamin Goldman, Jerome Groopman, Pauline Chen, Shelley Simon, and Margaret E. Mohrmann, to name only a few, believe that too often treatment goals are not clear; pain management becomes inconsistent, while medical practice ignores the person behind the illness.

Further, medical training and the medical system, to a large extent, deny the need for patient voice as a reflection of an important need to transition at life's end and in that denial often reduce life experiences to textbook interpretations. To confuse matters, a vast popular literature exists that promotes biotechnological advances that control human nature, while the same, narrow text often considers insightful stories emotional, *unscientific*, and superfluous. Consequently, patient narratives, as part of mainstream therapeutic practice, remain an initial concept (Rifkin 1983, 250).

Mainstream medical goals most often focus on disease resolution and dismiss the patient's pain as a necessary by-product. A physician's empathetic skills that consider a patient's pain, conflict, and acceptance rather than defiance improve medical practice because these skills enable and encourage transformation in both the physician and the patient. To be transformed is to perceive suffering *with ever-expanding vision* (Mohrmann 1995, 62).

Often over time with many patients, a physician may realize they have not enabled or appreciated personal suffering as a significant part of their medical practice. In *Final Exam, A Surgeon's Reflections on Mortality*, Pauline W. Chen discusses her fear, avoidance, learned responses, and inadequate approach with chronically ill patients during many years of medical practice.

Her pain of losing many *unknown* patients, that is, taking the human experience as seriously as anatomy or physiology, motivated her to write an anthology of her experiences dealing with pain. Chen's reappraisal of medical training enjoins a different perspective than her transplant surgeon training that focuses on precise, predictive analysis (Chen 2007, 1–10). She believes change in medical perceptions and goals may overcome medical training that often minimizes exchange and therefore separates rather than enjoins physicians to patients.

CONTEMPORARY THINKING, MEDICALIZATION, AND BEYOND

Psychological researchers tell us, "Pain is a subjective symptom, not directly verifiable by the physician. Nonetheless, the symptom of pain is of great clinical importance as it is often this complaint that motivates patients to seek health care" (Crooke, Rideout, and Browne 1984, 299). Pain is often associated with disability and is suggested as a major factor in affecting quality of life. Evidence indicates that pain relief becomes temporary and an incomplete response to existential suffering; therefore, the ensuing and ultimate isolation and alienation must be addressed as well (Crooke, Rideout, and Browne 1984).

As an independent anthropology researcher, Dr. David Morris speaks for his team of medical researchers on the management of pain and how that undertaking exactly relates to the person:

> Pain has a relationship with patient narrative—pain and narrative become interpersonal. Pain no longer consists of only a nervous system reaction but rather a specific cognitive-emotional attitude a patient embodies and needs to express. It is a matter of somehow expressing and describing experiences that normally retreat from language. (Morris 1991, 123)

Pain is a difficult word to describe. It becomes easy to understand why patients differ in ways and words to describe pain. The language of pain becomes a special way of desperately communicating, a way of developing a relationship with the outside world—of family, physician, and society—perhaps, particularly with society. How the patient communicates with their environment becomes *a cry for comfort* hoping for a reaction from contemporary culture. There is indeed, a language of its own, and this *pain language* perpetuates a *pained behavioral pattern* (Rey 1993, 335).

Persistent or chronic pain is the primary reason people seek medical care, yet current therapies are either inadequate for certain types of pain or cause intolerable side effects. Recently, pain neurobiologists have identified a number of cellular and molecular processes that lead to the initiation and maintenance of pain. Understanding these underlying mechanisms has given significant promise for the development of more effective, more specific pain therapies in the near future for physiological pain. Some researchers go as far as to say that pain is like a disease. However, you cannot predict pain by looking at MRI scans or an X-Ray (Rey 1993, 335).

An in-patient, Patrick (The INPUT program [for chronic pain sufferers] at St. Thomas's Hospital, London, UK) considers pain a dark and lonely place:

> It is not only to doctors that chronic pain patients find it difficult to articulate what they are experiencing, but to family and friends (and not even to them at times). The place this leaves them is often lonely and unreachable by those outside it. One sufferer described how he was unable to talk about his pain even to those closest to him. His experience of 'self' disintegrated and he withdrew so far he became trapped *in a dark and isolated space*. (Padfield 2003, 17)

THE SUBJECTIVE EXPERIENCE OF PAIN ENTRENCHED IN THE MEDICALIZATION OF SOCIETY

Why are there differences in reaction to and perception of the pain factor?

The answer is your brain decides its own priorities. Our reality is therefore filtered through culture, history, evolution, prior learning, in fact, anything that is relevant to you. One fact permeates our existence on this earth—humanity and pain are intertwined. As Arthur McGill has pointed out, our culture presents a dualistic conception of humanity and pain. If you have humanity, you have no pain. If there is pain, then there is no humanity, hence, the medicalization of the problem—to maintain humanity at all cost, "even if it means large doses of anesthetizing drugs" (Lammers and Verhey 1987, 247).

Evolution has taught us that danger signals and the perception of threat are high-value signals when discussing pain. Conditioned processing quickly takes over the functioning of the whole organism in somewhat of *a knee-jerk reaction*. Why does our brain get stuck in an automatic mode and make mistakes? The problem with chronic pain is that evolution was not such a good negotiator in resolving this error. Within our perceptual limitations, the most important decision your brain makes is, *Am I safe?* Do the sensations of pain relate to the evolutionary, primary instinct of safety first? Or has our evolved network of thinking and reacting evolved into a maze of perceived and debunked threats to the integrity of our well-being? (Haines 2015, 13).

In "Looking at Pain," in Padfield's *Perception of Pain*, Professor Hurwitz tells us that pain has driven people into the hands of doctors more often than any other symptom in human history. Our experience of pain is therefore foundational to medicine. So is recognition of the immensely varied ways we express and communicate it: silently in shivers, gazes, and winces and in the stretching, twisting writhing movements of the body; acoustically in shrieks, screams, or whimpers; onomatopoeically in sighs, moans, and groans; verbally in strangely figurative descriptions; and socially by withdrawal from the world (Padfield 2003, 7).

THE SUBTLE BUT DISTINCTIVE DIFFERENCES BETWEEN PAIN AND SUFFERING

What do we know today?

There is indeed a renewed interest in pain—the invisible epidemic, which has changed the role of physicians according to the demands and needs of the public. Formal education, such as the basic, first cycle of medical school education, still limits formal study, but postgraduate courses on pain are becoming more available. Physicians no longer feel righteous in allowing pain in patients—for the good, and there is, by all accounts, a painful crisis.

Acute pain is never good and needs an immediate, urgent response. Chronic pain becomes a completely different affair. We must closely analyze its underlying, ruminating causes and effects, its somatic origins—excessive nociceptive afferents and its neurophysiological and psychological causes.

THE TRAGIC RESPONSE TO PAIN

What are the true origins of human anguish and who are the victims? There are many psychosocial reasons for pain and despair. The challenge becomes ours to decide our values and exactly where our responsibility lies in protecting the vulnerable. Social science offers an application of cultural constructs such as the disenfranchised, gender inequality, transgender issues, drug addictions, sexual addictions, PTSD, the effect of physical, mental abuse, and common mental symptoms that affect behavior, just to name a few experiences that raise ethical issues concerning those who really suffer.

When approaching the symptoms of disease, the healthcare professional should realize that most people in pain tend to tell their life stories—according to the past, present, and future (Doyle 1992, 305). The healthcare professional, especially the physician, should own the role as one who genuinely hears—no, listens to and enters into—the story of the person in pain: to stand beside that person and let the story inform the response—the care plan.

CONCLUDING REMARKS

There is a real partnership between the physician and society now in realizing the importance of understanding pain to the best of our professional skills and human abilities. Hopefully, physicians and social partners work together toward wellness as well as social, long-term resilience by studying biocultural models thereby educating healthcare students to consider the entire person.

Medical humanists programs seated within therapeutic narratives reflect, embody, and enable the voices of vulnerable populations. The medical humanists who create spaces for healthcare professionals to enter into the narratives of vulnerable, pained populations aim to develop research questions for further study in response to unimaginable pain. Together, healthcare professionals with medical humanists learn to speak for those who cannot or will not speak for themselves. The next chapter invites the teachers of healthcare professionals to consider one model for learning to care for the entire person, to hear the voices of people in pain.

REFERENCES

Chen, Pauline W. 2007. *Final Exam*. New York: Knopf, Borzoi Books.

Crooke, J., E. Rideout, and G. Browne. March 1984. *The Prevalence of Pain in a General Population. Pain* 18 (3): 299–314.

Doyle, Derek. July 1992. "Have We Looked Beyond the Physical and Psychosocial?" *Journal of Pain and System Management* 7 (2): 302–311.

Gunderman, R. B. 1990. "Medicine and the Question of Suffering." *Second Opinion* 14: 15–25.

Haines, S. 2015. *Pain Is Really Strange*. New York: Jessica Kingsley.

Lammers, S. E., and A. Verhey, eds. 1987. *On Moral Medicine: Theological Perspectives in Medical Ethics*. Grand Rapids, MI: William B. Eerdmans.

Mohrmann, Margaret. 1995. *Medicine as Ministry: Reflections on Suffering, Ethics, and Hope*. New York: Pilgrim Press.

Morris, D. 1991. *The Culture of Pain*. Berkeley, CA: University Press.

Padfield, D. 2003. *Perceptions in Pain*. Manchester: Dewi Lewis.

Pellegrino, E. 2001a. "The Internal Morality of Clinical Medicine: A Paradigm for the Ethics of the Helping and Healing Professions." *Journal of Medicine and Philosophy* 26 (6): 559–79.

Pellegrino, E. 2001b. "Philosophy of Medicine: Should It Be Teleologically or Socially Constructed?" *Kennedy Institute of Ethics Journal* 11(2): 177–78.

Pernick, M. S. 1985. *A Calculus of Suffering: Pain, Professionalism and Anesthesia in 19th Century America*. New York: Columbia Press.

Rey, R. 1993. *The History of Pain*. Paris: Histoire de la Douleur.

Rifkin, Jeremy. 1983. *Algeny*. New York: Viking Press.

Stuckey, C. L., M. S. Gold, and X. Zhang. 2001. "Mechanisms of Pain." *Proceedings of the National Academy of Science of the United States of America* 98: 11845–11846.

Chapter 7

Epigogy: The Education of Humanity: The Psychology of Pain as It Affects the Human Condition

Gaetana Kopchinsky

We must understand the context of pain to comprehend social change and how those changes affect the human condition.

INTRODUCTION SEMESTER 1

1. Students should engage with other class participants (in order) to properly appreciate the complexities of the construct of pain. The class critiques visual aids such as graphics. In this way, each of us slowly absorb, understand, and share the definition of pain in contemporary society and discover how, specifically, that definition has evolved. The presentation involves a basic, rather lengthy, review of the history and literature of pain. The participants further accomplish the investigative task by assigning advanced readings, such as R. Rey's *The History of Pain* (1993), E. Scarry's *The Body in Pain* (1985) (certain assigned sections), and D. Morris's *The Culture of Pain* (1991).
2. The next step, as a group, is to discuss the meaning of self-knowledge as described in A. Siegel's *H. Kohut and The Psychology of the Self* (1978) and how that information relates to empathetic understanding of another person's suffering. The seminar community does this in several ways: (1) Discuss the meaning of personhood (its relational context), the true comprehension of which is essential to our studies because of the social trend toward patient-centered care. (2) Refer to each participant's degree of self-knowledge as *the entire person* behind the professional.

    In simple terms, *What is it we are looking for in ourselves (always in relation to another) in terms of our humanity?* The subject of personhood is a complex topic that involves an in-depth "unpacking" of the normative

ethics that surround our value system. In other words, the way we live every day, the choices we make, and how we cope with adversity all contribute to our character formation and the legacy of tradition we leave behind even in adversity. In some cases, this approach may conflict with a medicalized approach to pain.
3. In view of the previous introduction, the course review includes the following precepts. These principles are presented to the class for open discussion and debate to set the tone of our pedagogy.

   A. Medical ethics bases its scholarly concepts on an enduring reason and hope that medicine may connect technological discovery to nature in a symbiotic union rather than subject humankind to its methods. This type of natural philosophy and union seeks to define the essence of humankind in all its ways of achieving some type of harmony that scientific discovery ultimately should serve.
   B. Principles of ethical healing should guide technological advances to constitute a *better and worse* construct of care for the individual (as well as) that agencies should assess these changes as legitimate. The person behind the patient has worth beyond technological advance that includes an individual perception of a good life (Conrad and Gabe 1999, 505). (Included in that perception are the limits of our ability to sustain pain and suffering.)

   A good life is not defined by technology. The personal distinctions of value and solutions to ambiguities are difficult, require reflection, and cannot be bound to negotiation of our natural reasoning. A second ethical consideration becomes the question, "Who should decide what is real pain and how much pain is enough?"
   C. New technical insights often become standards to which we conform without regard for individuality in patient values. Collaborative social values become a powerful overriding mechanism as a means of scientific usefulness. These constructs of *functional* worth are always changing but the person within the patient never changes. According to Edmund Pellegrino, there remains a constant need for understanding and expression amid the particular changes illness brings to his or her life. Cultural contexts dictate each tradition, vote, and scientific endeavor and may shape scientific knowledge in the process.

   Those social ideologies advance theory as worthy or not. Knowledge, however, may no longer be viewed as a natural discovery, but rather as an ongoing utilitarian process that presumably serves human needs to maintain and extend life without necessarily a regard for the quality of that life that self-knowledge indeed promotes (Pellegrino 2001, 178). Only then, when people examine self-knowledge in terms of one's values, may they appreciate the fact many sufferers endure pain symptoms quietly because of superficial value systems, feelings of guilt, and low esteem. Consequently, their suffering remains hidden from society—even from partners and other family members.

4. As part of the didactic portion of the course, students and instructor examine the biopsychosocial differences in pain and the demarcations between acute and chronic pain as they know a contemporary definition and context. (Participants accomplish this by reviewing the normal guidelines about pain.) Conversation partners form small groups to explore what they, as individuals, consider real pain to be; its etiology and how that basic philosophy *fits* into a contemporary setting.

Course Description

The course curriculum is a comprehensive look at the innovative clinical interest in pain, the societal need to examine its cause and effect in terms of contemporary living. Throughout this course, students look at raw human suffering; its complex mental, emotional, and physical consequences; and how the impact/cost of distress may translate into dysfunctional behavior. Subjects explored through discussion, lecture, readings, and scholarly writing will include (not limited to) the following:

A. The basic definition of pain—differences in terms of individual experiences and perceptions (pain is covered under sub-section 4 in the Introduction).
B. How participants experience pain only as they internally interpret their universe.
C. Pain as illustrated in the arts; discussion of the *drama of pain*—as in works by Samuel Becket and others that describe the utilization of literature as a powerful voice to express pain.
D. Addictive behaviors as a faulty response to pain.
E. The effect of physical and mental abuse in terms of one's voice.
F. Uniting voices with bodies toward wellness.

Student Learning Outcomes

Students establish healthy traditions for contemporary living that includes techniques to (1) understand signs/symptoms of pain with the objective of a realistic path to wellness; (2) describe/articulate how pain has become medicalized as a dysfunction/disease by cultural influences within a position of change; (3) learn the pitfalls of drug addiction in terms of addiction as an invisible epidemic and the benefits of therapies such as the Drug Court Program; (4) and present an intelligent position on specific areas of pain pathology in terms of its effect on the human condition according to individual focus in the medical humanities program.

Practicum

Step 1: To begin, as a practical class exercise, visually observe the voiceless images of people in a deplorable, helpless situation (mental sanitarium Greece 1996—Island of Crete). These images are presented in slide formation from the professor's collected photographs to enhance student's learning experience and invite empathetic awareness.

Step 2: Advance instructional experience by walking students through a virtual tour of various contemporary settings: observe graphic displays of asylums, INPUT program art displays for outpatients (St. Thomas Hospital, UK) with chronic pain and PTSD (https://www.researchgate.net/project/Perceptions-of-Pain), as well as drug court therapeutic narrative journals and expressive art work. The latter is prepared by drug court participants who are given various topics for narrative and creative expression (see https://njcourts.gov/public/drugcourt/drugcourt2018.html or https://www.youtube.com/watch?v=_Q6Zk0L5Q8Y). Students explore how personal, self-knowledge narrative works pertain to the medical humanities.

Step 3: Participants then discuss graphically displayed behavioral symptoms of trauma with focus on PTSD. Either the instructor or the students create a slide presentation of the symptoms experienced by people suffering from PTSD. Symptoms resulting from pain, trauma, and abuse include but are not limited to extreme rage, short tempers, isolation, numbness, alcohol and drug use, memory problems, lack of concentration, low self-esteem, being startled, lack of sleep, and lack of appetite.

The class looks at a history of evolving scenarios which depict victims seeking refuge and peace of mind from raw suffering and others who continually have chronic pain. They do this by reviewing the literature of the suffering body through the lens of Susannah Mintz and other authors, such as Rita Charon, Kathryn Montgomery, Guy Micco, Edmund Pellegrino, Suzanne Poirier, and Johanna Shapiro (Mintz 2013). Those pundits describe through prose and relational narratives the symptoms and evolution of the inner conflicts that accompany illness. Students examine the themes and thick description of the rhetoric for clues of an evolving attempt toward some degree of wellness.

Case Study Exercise

During this second stage of the instructional process, seminar partners examine numerous examples of PTSD, as well as patient stories of extreme mental, physical, and emotional suffering. Students will look at acute and chronic pain situations as told in the history of pain, and review the etiology of pain's definition in a context that has changed over the last few centuries in terms of quality. Students then correlate readings to case studies as described previously; connect this information to the history of pain as told in oral discourse; and refine its etiology in terms of its present definition into a composite picture of pain as a contemporary societal plague.

Partners discuss Kaufman's (1986) work *The Ageless Self* work on the themes and value systems developed over the life span of pain sufferers. Following Kaufman's model, the instructor may offer their template of their discovery of lifetime themes and values to class participants. The instructor provides an in-depth slide presentation on the many *faces of pain* that offer graphic representations that expand psychological, inner conflict and further define these constructs of mental, physical, and emotional suffering.

Students then focus on individual relational narratives that each student has prepared according to life experiences. As explained in an earlier curriculum exhibit, seminar partners engage each other, as a next step, to *connect the dots* between case studies, the literature read, and their own unique perspectives. Participants do this by sharing notes and short narratives leading to new understanding of the experience of pain.

Then, the class discusses individual relational narratives (Cavarero 2000) in order to determine how each of us best processes a better sense of self-knowledge in relation to diversity. They refer, in this way, to the humanistic and reflective side of medicine—since we have as humans a relational impulse to communicate these experiences and feelings.

The discussion on voice and power will further detail the situations when that relational need is taken away by force. Therefore, any ensuing narrative/discourse becomes interpersonal. As students of the relational narrative, they discover that the pain sufferer craves recognition and a voice as a coping strategy. Class discourse reflects the themes and language people as pain sufferers express in literature like the therapeutic narrative.

Toward the end of the case study exercise, students and instructor, studying different contemporary authors, analyze the method with which they describe how pain has become medicalized in contemporary society as a dysfunction/disease by cultural influences. Examples of these authors are D. Morris, E. Cassell, R. Rey, and D. Padfield. They then discuss how culture not only influences but also dictates responses to pain—silence, anger, submission, and how we move toward a resilience and wellness—and discover a method of coping by corrective action versus inaction and despair within a cultural context.

Part 2: Second Semester of Learning: The Structure of Discourse and Its Influence on Language

1. *The Structures of Language*. The language of any civilization, for example, in Western culture, is usually contextualized by a specific time and place. Students consider the following: People cannot say everything at once, nor does every event occur at once. They look at the elements and

categories of time of the narrating. They do this because the temporal elements provided by the narrator provide coordinates and give life to the narrative's significance. So, too, personal stories of chronic suffering—whether mental, physical, or emotional—are constructed by character formation and placed in the context of a situation.

A very important part of the pedological experience becomes the time and place of the oral discourse. The reason is by attributing a contextual basis for the dialogue, seminar contributors provide meaning and voice to the afflicted population by way of a medium or having an external world as a hopeful promise (Mintz 2013, 95).

2. *Imagination as the Road Map to Language:* Human beings tell their ideas to others by the design and portrayal of human emotions, pain, and suffering. Creative thinking becomes the natural progression at this learning moment during the seminar. Thinking *outside of the box* in terms of narration offers a pivotal time in space wherein students uncover a character formation which begs the question of what matters most to us and the reason for our way of thinking. Trauma as the result of physical dysfunction and suffering offer that psychological construct memorialized by our writing. As a class, the consideration of stories move the seminar toward a discussion of Gretchen A. Case and Guy Micco's *Imagination Takes the Stage: Readers' Theater in a Medical Context. Journal for Learning through the Arts, 2 (1)*, 2006 (https://doi.org/10.21977/D92110072).

3. *The Turn toward Narrative Knowledge from Autobiographical Narration.* The class now focuses on autobiographical narrating, where the narrative brings its hero to the point where the narrative awaits him/her, where the two *hypostases* might meet and finally merge. (The gap between the hero and the narrator no longer exists.) No longer is the pain sufferer a victim, but rather a hero overcoming insurmountable obstacles. *Autobiographers are performers of sorts, choosing to display themselves within the parameters of the texts* (Mintz 2013, 11).

4. *How Are Voice, Narration, and Ethics Interconnected?* Narration becomes normative ethics in terms of describing how we live—our values based upon what matters the most to us and why. The instructor conducts a workshop environment [over several class sessions] by exchanging student writing samples to reflect this thought process.

5. *Narrative Knowledge.* Not only medicine but also nursing, law, history, philosophy, anthropology, sociology, religious studies, and government have recently realized the importance of narrative knowledge. What exactly is narrative knowledge?

Narrative knowledge is what one uses to understand the meaning and significance of stories through cognitive, symbolic, and affective means. This kind of knowledge provides, a rich, resonant comprehension of a singular person's situation as it unfolds in time, whether in such texts as novels, newspaper stories, movies, and scripture or in such life settings as court rooms, battlefields, marriages, and illnesses. (Humanitas 2015, 211)

Clearly, we observe a domain of knowledge gathered in a relational context—a situation of revelation about human beings. As literary critic R. W. B. Lewis writes, "Narrative deals with experiences, not with propositions" (Humanitas 2015, 211). Unlike its complement, logico-scientific knowledge, through which a detached and replaceable observer generates or comprehends replicable and generalizable notices, narrative knowledge leads to local and understandings about one situation by one participant or observer. Logico-scientific knowledge attempts to illuminate the universally true by transcending the particular; narrative knowledge attempts to illuminate the universally true by revealing the particular—the particulars of our topic. Narrative considerations probe the intersubjective domains of human knowledge and activity; those aspects of life that are enacted in the relation between two persons. Literary scholar Barbara Hernstein Smith [quoted in Humanitas] defines narrative discourse as "someone telling someone else that something else happened," emphasizing narrative's requirement for a teller and a listener, a writer and a reader, a communion of sort (ibid.).

The narratively competent reader or listener realizes that the meaning of any narrative—a novel, a textbook, a joke—must be judged in the light of its narrative situation: Who tells it? Who hears it? Why and how is it told? The narratively skilled reader further understands that the meaning of a text arises from the ground between the writer and the reader. With narrative competence, multiple sources of local—and possibly contradicting—authorities replace master authorities; instead of being monolithic and hierarchically given, meaning is apprehended collaboratively, by the reader and the writer, the observer and the observed, the physician and the patient [in this case, the sufferer] (ibid.).

6. *Voice and Its Illustration: Connecting the dots—voice, the self, and narration.* According to S. Mintz, *The narrator's impulse to enumerate his pains, to suppress feeling and amplify talking, foregrounds language as the "medium for having a world"* (Mintz 2013, 95). Further, *Pain impels its own voicing or narration: it presumes, even depends on, being witnessed to give it coherent form* (Humanitas 2015, 211). Perhaps unexpectedly, Samuel Beckett, playwright (in Mintz's literature), profoundly suggests that *pain must be expressed to be made meaningful, that it resides within, rather than being inimical to, language. Pain is powerfully intersubjective, not only in the phenomenological sense of establishing relations between embodied subjects but also because it initiates a*

kind of storytelling that, in demanding to be read, moves outward from the self (Humanitas 2015, 211).

At this point of instruction, the class portrays the drama of this subject by presenting a scene of an author or their own design [in pairs] as a class exercise.

7. *The Drama of Pain and Samuel Beckett. Pain is elemental, a first principle of human experience and identity* (Humanitas 2015, 94). The class discusses the different types of literary portrayal of pain. For example, they examine a conventional construct in forms such as autobiographical staging of narrative prose. Then there is the *egotistical pain*, when authors embody their pain in startling imagery and metaphor and collisions of lyric pain in poetry (ibid., 10).

8. *The Definition of Pain Revisited.* There are differences and similarities in terms of individual perceptions of pain. Students consider how individuals experience of pain translates to how they internally interpret their respective universes. Students present an individual case history (in an organized fashion) of personal recollection and interpretation.

9. *The Role of the Medical Humanist: Seeking Out the Art of Those Who Do Not Have a Voice.* As a group of medical humanists, seminar participants examine the effect of history on the philosophy and values of medicine by looking at the history of medical ethics. They look at how a process of caring along with healing has emerged over time in an inconsistent pattern. Students and instructor look at the history of medical ethics, which is really a cultural context of the way we historically treat the suffering of others. They read *The History of Pain,* as chronologically depicted by Roselyne Ray.

However, students also lean heavily on the history of oral discourse and the stories of those pain victims who seek a way of expressing pain and how suffering has changed them and how the ethical portion of medicine has responded to these cries for help. As far as their empowerment as individuals, seminar members listen to the words of Eric Cassell—*The Nature of Suffering* (Cassell 2004). Turning then to how normative ethics are formed by everyday choices and coping skills as shown by history and authors such as Mintz (2013), *Hurt and Pain*, and Cavarero, *The Relational Narrative.* Seminar conversation gives close attention to how those choices shape values in everyday living.

Narrative becomes the shape of ethics—of how people treat each other, medically and otherwise.

10. *Pain in the Arts:* Students explore pain as illustrated in the arts in terms of this continuing human need for expression, yet feeling of isolation. Students reflect on the works of artists such as Da Vinci's depiction (Pain vs. Pleasure), D. Padfield's INPUT program of individuals with chronic pain, E. Munch ("The Scream"), just to name several artists who have depicted a *snapshot of pain and suffering.*

Semester 2 Learning Objectives

Dysfunctional Behaviors

Students examine dysfunctional behaviors as a response to pain and how that dysfunction becomes a contemporary societal problem. The breakdown of the human spirit becomes a primary focus of our education with the objective being the discovery of the best method of treatment for victims of mental, physical, and emotional abuse.

Social Injustice

Students become schooled in the social injustice or inequity experienced when the voice of a vulnerable human being is exposed yet dismissed. The consequence of physical and mental abuse on vulnerable populations as a distinct social injustice affects everyone; therefore, it remains the individual's responsibility to review conditions when she cannot have her voice heard. At this point, seminar partners read and reflect on some of the readings that highlight power used to inflict pain as presented in E. Scarry's *The Body in Pain* (1985).

Voice

Students examine and delineate how people unite their voices with their bodies toward wellness.

Relational Narrative

After further exploration of the relationship between A. Cavarero's (2000) work and student narratives, seminar participants establish a connection with the outside world. The relational narrative (as a means of forming identities and human connections) provides a portal between the inner self and the outside world. Conversation partners revisit the readings on self-psychology the readings of A. Siegel's *H. Kohut, The Ageless Self* (1996) and P. Homan's *The Ability to Mourn* (1989). Class enrichment proceeds through reflection and self-knowledge.

Ethics

The ethics that drive the treatment and management of acute and chronic pain surrounds us. The instructor provides an in-depth look at the ethical philosophy in pain management. Students discern the moral legacy and tradition by a critical reflection on the choices they make as they consider pain treatment and management. The sociological tenets of Max Weber as they relate to pain management and treatment inform student reflections.

The Transient Nature of the Human Condition

Students evaluate the rational and affective abilities to alter one's way of thinking as the source of the individual's willingness to face their or another's pain issues and suffering.

Perception of the Universe through Pain

Students meet the challenges that the subject of neuroplasticity (discussion on the work of Moheb Costandi: *Neuroplasticity*, MIT 2016) presents to their way of thinking and reacting to crisis. For example, although the physiology of pain affects the human condition, through the regenerative aspects of neuroplasticity, the pain sufferer *reinvents* perception of the outside universe.

Exclusion

Students examine their biases about The Other particularly as those biases exclude socially people with disabilities, thus increasing awareness of who is considered a vulnerable population.

Pick a Disease—a Mental Disorder—a Disability

Students consider the following question: *have you ever felt the presence of pain in another human being without being able to see, hear, or touch them?* Students conceive and present an intelligent position on pain as it affects the human condition.

Assessments

Students and instructor evaluate learning outcomes for students through a self-assessment synthesis. The self-assessment synthesis analyzes a seminar participant's ability to determine *where we are in plotting/achieving our own individuation [self-growth]* as follows:

a. Purpose of our inquiry—in pursuing the ethics surrounding acute and chronic pain
b. Identity—determining where our interest fits within our own character formation

We create that unique identity with an examination of the following:

c. Values
d. Interests
e. Skills
f. Knowledge
g. Experiences (which include outreach community involvement)

In addition, a needs assessment for this type of learning will follow these guidelines in terms of *where do we go from here?*

World Needs

Students in their assessment synthesis evaluate their role as medical humanists who write for health, emotion, and freedom and provide a therapeutic writing program for the chronically ailing so that they also realize emotional and physical health and freedom (Humanitas 2015, 124).

Student assessment synthesis also reflects their abilities to collaborate as skilled readers, writers, observers, patients, and physicians to understand the meaning of pain in terms of how suffering affects the human condition.

Assessment synthesis also evaluates a student's ability and desire to pursue the ethical complications of pain among newborn, children, and young adults as vulnerable populations.

Finally, the seminar is a transfer learning, skill-based curriculum that includes interpretation, critical thinking, problem solving, ethical thinking, qualitative reasoning and collaboration, and oral, interpersonal, and written communication.

Exhibit A (Gaetana A. Kopchinsky, excerpts from *Negotiation with Death*, ProQuest, 2011)

Introduction: The following exhibit presents a model for a narrative that gives voice to the lives of pain sufferers. The narrative represents qualitative research, the data that a student draws from the person's experience as a patient in a medicalized society. Each student enters into an active listening relationship with a patient, observing respectfully the individual's behavior. That compassionate observation opens a world of insights into the person behind the patient. In addition, that descriptive narrative of a life observed directly informs a care plan for victims of acute and chronic pain.

Narrative Analysis as a Psychosocial Tool in Clinical Care of Acute and Chronic Pain Victims

Background: How do students make sense of observations? How do they synthesize the data in the conversations with the person behind the patient, using those interpretations and qualitative reasoning to relate to others?

A. *Observations* are a major means of collecting data in qualitative research. It offers a firsthand account of the situation under study and, when combined with interviewing and document analysis, allows for a holistic interpretation of the pain sufferers—in this case, the patient's story. It is the technique of choice because behavior can be observed firsthand. This becomes an important point since—that information is a primary source.

B. *The study of behavior* is only half the process because observations must be recorded in as much detail as possible to form the database for the analysis. That analysis must be weaved into a story that encompasses a curative plan of action.
C. *Field notes* include descriptions, direct quotations, and observer comments. Specifically, since this methodology has a large ethnographic component, we maintained *a fieldwork journal*—an introspective record of field experience. This experience includes ideas, thoughts about the research method itself. Such traumatic experiences include personal reactions to patient and family interactions.
D. *Listening, which actively and compassionately responds to the person* who is the patient, is crucial both to analyzing the data and to composing the narrative—the voice of the person in pain.

The following narrative tool aids students in creating and organizing an analysis feature to their studies. Each section is labeled and defined to facilitate shaping the qualitative analysis. The module is specifically designed to detail emotional, mental, and physical elements of the pain sufferer's experiences. So, its uniqueness comes from both an analysis and a synthesis.

Section I: Design and Structure of Research Module in Acute/Chronic Care Cases

The architecture is defined strictly in terms of establishing the context of *a world of pain* according to the sufferer and their experience.

A. *Domains and Definitions:* (a) Experience—a pain sufferer's unique reaction and navigation within a cultural context; (b) Opinion—individual perception of the social construct in terms of the medicalization of pain; (c) Values—what matters most to the pain sufferer and why; and (d) Knowledge—how the patient interprets and retains, utilizes his or her relational communication for personal use.
B. *Eligibility Criteria:* pain sufferers.

Section II: Organization—How Best to Group the Data We Obtain

The conditions to administer the module are usually clustered according to the social conditions/environment in which pain sufferers reside. This same individual (person behind the patient), in attempt to establish some voice, may express topics such as family disruption, role resource disparity, role reformation, social withdrawal, or a damaged sense of self-transforming dynamics.

Section III: How to Introduce and Administer the Module

During class discussions, participants establish parameters for obtaining consent, proper forms, and protocol to proceed.

Section IV: Tracking the Observation

- Pay attention to detail. Encourage the patient/person's thoughts, feelings, and experiences
- Shift from a large picture focus to a specific person, interaction, or activity in terms of clinical care—such as the INPUT program versus the output of the relational narrative.
- Look for key words in the person's remarks that will stand out later. What recurs?
- Concentrate on the first and last remarks in each conversation.
- Mentally play back remarks and scenes during breaks in observation.

Write down as close as one can a verbatim account of the conversation as soon as one can following the meeting.

Section V: Understanding the Reason to Develop a Profile—A Character Formation of How Pain Affects the Human Condition

Section VI: Using the Profile to Develop Themes of Importance

Note that at this point seminar participant should discuss software programs (such as Dedoose; reference https://www.dedoose.com/) to analyze different defining themes of patients suffering from chronic pain. Include a cultural context to refine the character formation and further qualify the quality of life as part of one's study.

CASE STUDIES

a. Verbal description of the setting, the people, the issues, the activities. (What do you see?)
b. Note direct quotations or at least the substance of what people said about coping skills, attitude toward the medicalization of the problem.

Section VII: Administration of the Profile

Form individual discussion groups to share creative approaches to using the *tool* most effectively.

Section VIII

Within each dimension, three kinds of information are gathered from respondents in order to clarify their overall experience within a social construct:

- *Evaluation*—researcher's measurement of actual status or circumstance of person's physical, mental, and emotional well-being
- *Realization*—locus of inner control—coping skills reconditioning cognitive behavior—neuroplasticity
- *Value*—degree to which a given dimension has an impact on overall quality of life

Each dimension is defined by the patient's perception or experience—not the *judgment* of caregivers (family or professional). The definitions for the dimensions and examples of items for each category are shown in the following:

Attitude Indices Worksheet: Characteristics of which students should be mindful in our observations.

Symptoms of Severe Cases of Acute and Chronic Pain and Trauma: Experience of physical discomfort associated with progressive illness and the perceived level of distress. One critical point to remember is that often less pain medication is required when a person is being provided care in a competent, gentle manner. Some symptoms of acute pain are restlessness, agitation, anxiety, confusion, fever, hemorrhaging, perspiring, nausea and/or vomiting, decreased eating and drinking, pain, skin wounds, fungal infections, topical infections, sore mouth/candidiasis (the most common type of yeast infection), shortness of breath, seizures, noisy moist breathing, incontinence or retention, jerking, twitching, and plucking. What is the best course of action?

Certain concepts to consider, which are *the road signs*, are the following:

- I feel sick, alone, and forgotten versus I am at peace with my condition.
- Pain and physical discomfort overshadow any opportunity for enjoyment, peace, or closure.

Function

The perceived ability to perform the accustomed functions and activities of daily living, experienced in relation to life expectations.

Assessment Tool

The following provides guidance for both understanding and the topics of interest that the interviewer should consider.

Scale of Information

Values for assessment are assigned points according to indications of affect: position, presence, gaze, and behavior as follows:

1. Shows aimlessness; shows isolation, complete negation, shame, despair, resistance;
2. Rarely does anything to communicate;
3. Barely communicates but talks about some experience; no connection; wants to get done with the interview;
4. Talks about no social subject to any great extent; some explanation of values and life;
5. Talks mostly about values and experience; talks with a clear explanation of personal experience and expression of salient values for full completion. Three key areas of relevance here are identifiability, autonomy, and spirituality.

Points are allowed for repetition of behavior or words to calibrate a Likert scale from 6 to 1:

Themes: Identity/confusion 6–1
Autonomy/shame 6–1
Spirituality/despair 6–1
Closure/resistance 6–1

a. Timing (when the interaction took place)—Sharon Kaufman's keynote quality
b. Style—Sharon Kaufman's keynote quality
c. Affect—Sharon Kaufman's keynote quality

Common Characteristics of Expression

1. Resistance
2. Closure
3. Expression of love
4. Expression or need for spirituality
5. Expression or need for self-esteem and acceptance
6. Ability to communicate experiences and values
7. Expression or need for *Letting go* of the material world

With each category of relevant *life experience* and for continuity of *self*, three dimensions of observation are evaluated toward scoring in order to elucidate their overall experience:

Evaluation—subjective dimension of actual status or circumstances.
Realization—degree of control of actual circumstances.
Value—degree to which a given dimension has an impact on overall quality of life.

The scale relates to the following: very important; somewhat important; not very important; not important at all; not sure; no response.

From Observations: Topics That Reflect Personal Concerns

a. Will I ever be *whole* again?
b. Honest answers from your doctor; honest answers from your family.
c. Comfort from religious/spirituality.
d. Visiting with family.
e. Having healthcare professionals and members of community visit.
f. Narrative competence in expressing pain: voice.
g. Writing a letter to a friend.
h. Understanding treatment.
i. Spending time reflecting.
j. Having as little pain as possible.

Following are *identity triggers* to attend to that are included in personal reflections and self-knowledge:

a. I want to walk; I want to go to church, I want to sing again.
b. I can do other things despite my condition.
c. My happiness with life depends upon being lively and free. I cannot accept my situation.

Interpersonal Dimensions

The patient's degree of investment in personal relationships and the perceived quality of one's relations with family and friends.

a. Is this person able to say important things to people who have had significance in the past? Is this person able to express their feelings about pain/trauma?
b. Does this person spend as much time as possible with family and friends?
c. Does the person being assessed have close relationships?

Psychosocial and spiritual markers are indications of a social construct, all of which contribute to character formation:

a. Is there a perceived (any) purpose to this person' life as he or she suffers?
b. Is this person able to transcend suffering and see something or someone beyond physical, emotional, and mental pain?
c. Is this person at peace and feel some measure of inner control?

d. Is this person hopeful in some way or is there only the sense of despair?
e. What nourishes a sense of value: sense of self-esteem; prayer, religion, personal faith, relationship with others?
f. Do their beliefs help (them cope) with their anxiety and with their pain, and with achieving peace?

Finally, one needs to assess how well the patient's spiritual needs are being met: (a) Do the healthcare providers listen? (b) Is this person able to express or develop their spirituality through prayer, reflections, images of heritage, religious or spiritual readings, rituals such as anointing or Communion, connection to others including God?

Case Study Identifiers as Raw Material for Unique Themes

The values and ideals of human behavior that represent structural factors toward identity are: achievement, success, productivity, work, progress, social usefulness, forgiveness, restitution, individual initiative, and spirituality.

Observation: informants reflect individual expressions of widely held ideals of human behavior.

Identifiers: perception, language, ability to connect, range of ability to transition through natural means other than technology that include perception, social connection; attitude behavior, language, and sense of spirituality.

Last Topic of the semester: Pain Management for People with Serious Illness in the Context of Opioid Use Disorder Epidemic—The NATIONAL Academy of Science, Engineering and Medicine (2019).

1. A seminar symposium on the opioid crisis:

    Resources: How to address what clinicians should do with a patient who has chronic pain, serious illness, and substance abuse. Notes from http://nap.edu/25435 (The National Academic Press).
    Pain Management for People with Serious Illness in the Context of the Opioid Use Disorder Epidemic Proceedings of Workshop (2019).

2. Organic pain has identifiable, *legitimate* causes such as bone metastases, degenerative disc disease, or inflammatory conditions and other types of pain idiopathic pain disorder. The message from the pain literature is clear that the distinction is not meaningful because chronic pain is not a symptom but rather a disease, regardless of the initial source of pain (Merlin 2019, 47). As a result, the idea that *organic pain* automatically

merits treatment with opioids no longer holds true. Several output topics are given here:

a. Quality of care
b. Comorbid issues in terms of drug abuse
c. N. J. Drug Court Program/Therapeutic Narrative

RECOMMENDED RESOURCES FOR COURSE USE

Augustine. 2007. *Confessions*. New York: Barnes and Noble.
Autobiography of St. Theresa. 1926. North Carolina: TAN Books.
Butler, J. P. 2005. *Giving an Account of Oneself*. New York: Fordham University Press.
Case, G. A., and G. Micco. 2006. "Imagination Takes the Stage: Readers' Theater in a Medical Context." *Journal for Learning through the Arts* 2 (1).
Cassell, E. 2004. *The Nature of Suffering and the Goals of Medicine*. New York: Oxford Press.
Cavarero, A. 2000. *The Relational Narrative*. New York: Routledge.
Chen, Pauline. W. 2007. *Final Exam*. New York: Knopf, Borzoi Books.
Conrad, P., and J. Gabe. 1999. "Introduction: Sociological Perspectives on the New Genetics: An Overview." *Sociology of Health and Illness*, 21 (5): 505.
Costandi, M. 2016. *Neuroplasticity*. Cambridge, MA: MIT Press.
Crooke, J., E. Rideout, and G. Browne. 1984. "The Prevalence of Pain in a General Population." *Pain* Mar 18 (3): 299–314.
Dolan, B., ed. 2015. *Humanitas: Readings in the Development of the Medical Humanities*. California: University of California.
Doyle, D. 1992. "Have We Looked beyond the Physical and Psychosocial?" *Journal of Pain and System Management* 7 (2): 302–11.
Eliot, T. S. 1915. *The Love Song of J. Alfred Prufrock,* Stanza XIV. In *Poetry: A Magazine of Verse at the Instigation of Ezra Pound*. https://www.poetryfoundation.org/articles/70239/the-love-song-of-j-alfred-prufrock-turns-100
Frankl, Viktor. 1946. *Man's Search for Meaning*. New York: Beacon Press.
Gunderman, R. B. 1990. "Medicine and the Question of Suffering." *Second Opinion* 14: 15–25.
Haines, S. 2015. *Pain Is Really Strange*. New York: Jessica Kingsley.
Homans, P. 1989. *The Ability to Mourn*. Chicago, IL: University of Chicago Press.
Kaufman, S. 1986. *The Ageless Self*. Madison, WI: University of Wisconsin Press.
Kopchinsky, G. A. 2011. *Negotiation with Death*. Ann Arbor, MI: University of Michigan.
Lammers, S. E., and A. Verhey, eds. 1987. *On Moral Medicine: Theological Perspectives in Medical Ethics*. Grand Rapids, WI: William B. Eerdmans.
Merlin, J. 2019. National Academies of Sciences, Engineering, and Medicine. 2019. *Pain Management for People with Serious Illness in the Context of the Opioid Use Disorder Epidemic: Proceedings of a Workshop*. Washington, DC: The National Academies Press. https://doi.org/10.17226/25435.

Mintz, S. 2013. *Hurt and Pain*. New York: Bloomsbury.

Mohrmann, Margaret. 1995. *Medicine as Ministry: Reflections on Suffering, Ethics, and Hope*. New York: Pilgrim Press.

Morris, D. 1991. *The Culture of Pain*. Berkeley, CA California University Press.

Mother Agnes of Jesus. 2010. *The Story of a Soul*. Charlotte, NC: Saint Benedict Press.

Padfield, D. 2003. *Perceptions in Pain*. Manchester, UK: Dewi Lewis.

Pellegrino, E. 2001. "Philosophy of Medicine: Should It Be Teleologically or Socially Constructed?" *Kennedy Institute of Ethics Journal* 11 (2): 177–78.

Pernick, M. S. 1985. *A Calculus of Suffering: Pain, Professionalism and Anesthesia in 19th Century America*. New York: Columbia Press.

Rando, Oliver. 2018. "Can We Really Inherit Trauma?" *New York Times*, December 11, D3.

Rey, R. 1993. *The History of Pain*. Paris: Histoire de la Douleur.

Rifkin, Jeremy. 1983. *Algeny*. New York: Viking Press.

Scarry, E. 1985. *The Body in Pain*. New York: Oxford Press.

Siegel, A. 1996. *Heinz Kohut, The Psychology of the Self*. New York: Routledge Press.

Stuckey, C. L., M. S. Gold, and X. Zhang. 2001. "Mechanisms of Pain." *Proceedings of the National Academy of Science of the United States of America* 98: 11845–846.

Chapter 8

Epilogue

Philip C. Scibilia

Reforming medical ethics and medical humanities education should build on foundations put in place over the last four decades. Medical educators now appreciate that human values must complement science in education. Medical ethics, humanities, humanistic skills, and professional behavior in medical education have been progressively emphasized and added since 1970. The changes occurred in two time periods—the 1970–1999 (civil rights and post-Tuskegee) period for medical schools and the 2000–present period for both medical schools and residencies. Our current period focuses on competencies (i.e., outcomes) of education, in which ethics and humanism play a central role.

The teaching of medical ethics is now a common element of the U.S. medical school curriculum and, indeed, is a required preclinical educational element. Present teaching programs require training not only in medical ethics but also in skills in medical humanism and professionalism that develop young doctors so that they achieve the general competencies expected in their residency education.

But medical ethics teaching today is often consigned to *bull sessions*—discussion groups on topical issues with a general sprinkling of those discussions during the four-year curriculum. That ethical pedagogy is not uniformly integrated into the rest of the curriculum (or across medical schools), which can make its relevance questionable to students and professors. This method of teaching ethics is not comprehensive. It mainly attends to anecdotes rather than the underlying principles and reasoning that should guide humanistic clinical care, and enjoys no sustained monitoring by individual faculty.

There is a need for the development of a standardized curriculum integrating scientific reasoning with humanities-based reasoning as presented in the chapters of this book—and called the *art and culture of medicine*. The curriculum's goal should be to build on one's cultural and philosophic background to inform one's role as a physician-scientist. The emerging physician-scientist could thereby acknowledge and use humanities-based reasoning in the humane care of his or her patients.

This curriculum should be distinct from any college experience of didactics that are detached from clinical relevance. Instead, this curriculum would emphasize clinical humanities linked to patient care and the professional formation of medical students, so that the student's reasoning and manner would be broadened. The humane care of the patient is the ultimate mandated goal. The proposed curriculum should have four components: argument-based reasoning in medical ethics, narrative-based reasoning in literature, creative reasoning in the fine arts, and historical reasoning in learning from the past to uncover hidden assumptions and biases.

We have focused on a few of the contemporary issues challenging medical education and practice. As science and medicine continue to advance, new issues are constantly being raised, for example, in neuroscience, bioengineering, and nanotechnology. Some of these emerging sciences and technologies may pose genuinely new questions for bioethics; others can be characterized as *old wine in new wineskins*. Controversy over those new questions is inevitable: as bioethicists identify and analyze new issues, they frame the debates of the twenty-first century.

About the Authors

Katie Grogan, DMH, MA, is associate director of the Master Scholars Program in Humanistic Medicine and Adjunct Instructor in the Division of Medical Humanities at the New York University School of Medicine.

Kirk Johnson, DMH, teaches at Seton Hall University in South Orange, New Jersey. He teaches courses in bioethics, global issues, philosophy, and religion. He is a member of the American Society of Bioethics and Humanities and the New York Academy of Medicine. He serves as a member of the Atlantic Health Systems Bioethics Committee.

Jeanne Kerwin, DMH, is a nationally certified consultant for healthcare ethics with thirty-five years of bedside experience with patients and families in acute and long-term care settings. She is a speaker at state and national levels and is affiliated with Atlantic Health System and Drew University in New Jersey.

Gaetana Kopchinsky, DMH, is a professor at Drew University's Caspersen Graduate School. She is a philanthropist, writer, humanist, and mentor of underprivileged and exceptional elementary, undergraduate, and graduate students. She has published a number of articles on contemporary clinical physician-patient issues.

Dominic P. Scibilia, PhD, MEd, Emeritus Associate Professor in religious studies in secondary and university education.

Philip C. Scibilia, DMH, MA, MLitt, is adjunct professor at Fordham University's Institute of International Humanitarian Affairs, and past Associate Professor and Director of the Graduate Program of Medical Humanities Caspersen School Graduate Studies at Drew University.

www.ingramcontent.com/pod-product-compliance
Lightning Source LLC
Chambersburg PA
CBHW030147240426
43672CB00005B/304